Alcoholism and Sexual Dysfunction: Issues in Clinical Management

Alcoholism and Sexual Dysfunction: Issues in Clinical Management

David J. Powell
Editor

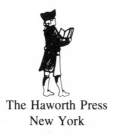

The Haworth Press
New York

Alcoholism and Sexual Dysfunction: Issues in Clinical Management has also been published as *Alcoholism Treatment Quarterly*, Volume 1, Number 3, Fall 1984.

The Haworth Press, Inc., 28 East 22 Street, New York, NY 10010

Library of Congress Cataloging in Publication Data
Main entry under title:

Alcoholism and sexual dysfunction.

"Has also been published as Alcoholism treatment quarterly, volume 1, number 3, fall 1984"—
Includes bibliographies.
1. Alcoholics—Sexual behavior. 2. Psychosexual disorders. I. Powell, David J. II. Alcoholism treatment quarterly. [DNLM: 1. Alcoholism—complications. 2. Sex Disorders—etiology. 3. Sex Disorders—therapy. 4. Sex Behavior. 5. Alcoholism—therapy. WM 274 A3498]
RC565.A4455   1984   616.86'1   84-12764
ISBN 0-86656-365-2

Alcoholism and Sexual Dysfunction: Issues in Clinical Management

Alcoholism Treatment Quarterly
Volume 1, Number 3

CONTENTS

Contributors

David J. Powell, Ph.D., CAC. President, Education and Training Programs, Inc. Diplomate in the International Academy of Professional Counseling and Psychotherapy. Certified Alcoholism Counselor. Certified Sex Therapist (AASECT).

Barry W. McCarthy, Ph.D. Professor, The American University. Psychologist, Washington Psychological Center. Chairperson, Admissions Committee, Society of Sex Therapy and Research (SSTAR). Diplomate in Clinical Psychology.

Sandra R. Leiblum, Ph.D. Professor, New Jersey College of Medicine and Dentistry, Sexual Counseling Service, Rutgers University.

Raymond C. Rosen, Ph.D. Professor, New Jersey College of Medicine and Dentistry, Sexual Counseling Service, Rutgers University.

Mildred Apter-Marsh, Ph.D. Private practice in California. Consultant to the Phoenix Alcohol and Drug Abuse Programs. Secretary of the U.S. Consortium for Sexology. Certified Sex Therapist by the American College of Sexologists.

Robert W. Fuller, MA. Program Coordinator, Employee Assistance Program, U.S. Tobacco International. 14 years clinical experience in alcoholism and drug abuse programming.

Dana G. Finnegan, Ph.D., CAC. Director, Alcoholism Out-patient Program, East Orange General Hospital, East Orange, New Jersey. National Coordinator for the National Association of Gay Alcoholism Professionals.

David Cook, CSW. Psychotherapist in private practice in New York.

Jerry Edelwich, MSW. Assistant Professor, Manchester Community College, Manchester, Ct. Co-author of *Burnout: Stages of Disillusionment in the Helping Professions,* and *Sexual Dilemmas for the Helping Professional.* Certified Reality Therapist.

Archie Brodsky, BA. Professional writer specializing in medicine, psychology and human services. Co-author of *Burnout*, and *Sexual Dilemmas for the Helping Professional*, and author of *Love and Addiction*, and *Medical Choices, Medical Chances*.

David E. Smith, M.D. Founder and Medical Director of Haight-Ashbury Free Medical Clinic, San Francisco, California.

Foreword

The editorial board of *Alcoholism Treatment Quarterly* is delighted to present this special issue of the Journal on alcoholism and sexual dysfunction. We have long recognized that a variety of sexual disorders are endemic in recovery from alcoholism and other drug dependencies, and the nature of such disorders have been well documented. However, very little information is available on specific treatment methodologies for sexual problems in recovery. In this light, this issue of *ATQ*, edited by David Powell, Ph.D., is a landmark in the field.

The material is of special interest to all clinicians who work with recovering alcoholics and their families: Alcoholism counselors, physicians, social workers, psychologists, clergy, nurses, and rehabilitation counselors. The material is also of special interest to sex therapists who are often undereducated about the nature of alcoholism and the process or recovery from the illness.

As Powell notes in the preface,

> As alcoholism workers become increasingly involved with sexual problems in their clients, there will be a growing awareness and knowledge in the areas of clinical practice, research, and policy. Our awareness of the interrelationship of sexual problems and alcoholism may be old, but our knowledge of what to do about it and our commitment to treat both problems is emerging and skills are developing.

This issue of *Alcoholism Treatment Quarterly* is a major contribution to that effort.

Bruce Carruth, Ph.D.
Editor

xi

Preface

The interrelationship of alcohol use and sexual activity has been established for milleniums. The awareness that alcohol abuse impacts on sexual problems has been alluded to by Shakespeare, medical practitioners and, more recently, alcoholism professionals. It was not until the mid to late 1970s that the alcoholism field universally recognized that alcoholism can result in sexual problems such as impotence, ejaculatory incompetence, inhibited sexual desire, and anorgasmia. In fact, the rule in dealing with an alcoholic should be: if you see one, look for the other. If a person is alcoholic, he/she will probably experience some sexual difficulties.

Sexual problems in alcoholics are multi-faceted, impacting on all aspects of functioning. Because it may have an organic etiology, general medical practice as well as urology, gynecology, neurology, etc., may be involved. The frequency of physical trauma, such as rape and incest, means that legal professionals are included in the treatment process. The psychological and relational impact of sexual problems of alcoholics involves social work, psychiatry, clinical psychology, and all aspects of counseling. It is truly a problem with a multi-dimensional and interdisciplinary focus.

Alcoholism counseling, with its dual interest in achieving sobriety and general emotional and relationship health, can and should play a significant role in responding to the sexual problems of alcoholics. Alcoholism professionals are in a unique position to insure that other disciplines are sensitive to the particular needs of the alcoholic and that services are provided in a manner that confronts the primary problem of alcoholism and enhances the person's potential for sobriety.

Alcoholism counselors can also advocate for the creation of special intervention programs for the alcoholic, his sexual partner, and other individuals such as family members and victims of sexual assault occurring under the influence of alcohol. The role alcoholism professionals play in dealing with sexual problems of alcoholics is limited only by our lack of knowledge, experience, and clinical skills.

There should be an overlapping and complementary interaction between the field of alcoholism treatment and sex therapy. Sexologists are cognizant of the biological basis for sexual dysfunction in alcoholics, with alcohol ingestion as the major factor in the production of such problems. Alcoholism counselors are becoming aware that sexual dysfunctions can contribute to the initiation of alcohol problems and are a factor in the relapse of the patient, and thus that treatment of alcoholism should address sexual issues. Unfortunately, until very recently, this was as far as the fields went in carving out a complementary and mutual approach to treatment. For example, most alcoholism treatment programs provide just a brief lecture on sexual problems and may ask the patient on intake "How's your sex life?" That is the extent to which the problem is addressed.

Sex therapists have traditionally avoided dealing with the alcoholism issues or have not treated the alcoholic at all. In fact, there is a nationally recognized sex therapy program that requests their alcoholic patients to "simply discontinue drinking while in treatment."

Therefore, a closer relationship must be drawn between these fields. We view this collection of articles as an attempt to forge this relationship, combining input from sexologists and alcohologists. A Journal Edition devoted exclusively to the treatment of sexual problems in alcoholics is to date unique. Volumes have been written on the nature and extent of sexual problems in alcoholics, and textbooks published on general sex therapy approaches. Little has been written specifically addressing sex treatment approaches for alcoholics.

To illustrate the dearth of literature available, in searching for authors for this issue, the editor was informed by a number of noted sex therapists that they do not treat alcoholics or have little interest in writing on the subject. It was equally difficult to recruit alcohologists with credentials and experience in sex therapy. Several alcoholism counselors were "experts" on general sexuality; few were in sex counseling and therapy.

The goal of this Special Edition is to enhance awareness in both the sexology and alcoholism fields about the interrelationship of these problems and to encourage further cooperation. With this focus, the Journal should be of interest to both alcoholism counselors and sex therapists. This volume is not the exhaustive edition on the subject; it is an initial attempt to focus exclusively on therapy approaches with alcoholics.

There are several unresolved or unaddressed issues that remain. Questions still exist as to the physiological factors in sexual problems of alcoholic women, sexual dymorphism and alcoholism, biological factors of homosexuality in alcoholics, the commonality of similar drug groups, and the interactive effects of alcohol and other drugs on sexuality. Clinical issues remaining include sex treatment outcome studies with alcoholics, the appropriate stage of recovery to initiate sex counseling, recommended laboratory tests for differential diagnosis of sexual problems in alcoholics, the specific needs of single alcoholics, and the treatment issues for broad intimacy disorders. Finally, both the sexology and alcoholism fields need to examine their attitudes and information bases about the dual problem and develop their skills in treatment of alcoholism and sexual impairment in an objective and non-judgmental manner.

The contributions collected here represent the state of knowledge concerning sex therapy with alcoholics. They include reviews of the impact of alcoholism on sexual functioning, issues surrounding the professionals' response to treatment, and specific therapy models for alcoholism programs. Contributors have also addressed a number of clinical concerns including treatment of homosexuality in alcoholics and ethical issues for the alcoholism professional.

The first article by Sandra Leiblum, Ph.D., and Raymond C. Rosen, Ph.D., presents an overview of alcohol and alcoholism and its effects on human sexual response. Dr. Smith et al. discuss the broad treatment issues in alcoholism and the prevalence of sexual problems in alcoholic males and females. Barry McCarthy, Ph.D., examines the alcoholic's return to drinking as a result of erectile dysfunction. The third paper by Mildred Apter-Marsh, Ph.D., presents the most interesting and current research available on female alcoholic's sexual functioning. For the first time, special sexual problems at various stages of addiction and sobriety are compared. The implications of this research for treatment are addressed.

A critical stage in treatment is determining an accurate, complete differential diagnosis. Robert Fuller's chapter presents the various issues to be reviewed in assessment, laboratory and clinical tests to be performed, and the appropriate use of this information in determining a diagnosis.

David J. Powell, Ph.D., addresses the most prevalent sexual problem in male alcoholics: impotence. The PLISSIT model for treatment is presented as well as other diagnostic and therapy approaches.

A significant number of alcoholics are troubled with sexual identity concerns. Ego dystonic homosexuality is a significant issue to be addressed in alcoholism therapy. Therefore, Dana Finnegan's and David Cook's article on gays and lesbians is pivotal in understanding the treatment of sexual issues in homosexual alcoholics.

The final chapter is by Jerry Edelwich, M.S.W., and Archie Brodsky, B.A., on ethical concerns in treatment. As in any newly emerging field, the opportunity for abuse of skills and knowledge is always possible. Edelwich and Brodsky appropriately point out the limits in counseling for sexual problems and pitfalls clinicians may encounter.

The Journal concludes with a glossary of terminology and recommendations for further study and training.

As alcoholism workers become increasingly involved with sexual problems in their clients, there will be growing awareness and knowledge in the areas of clinical practice, research, and policy. Our awareness of the interrelationship of sexual problems in alcoholics may be old, but our knowledge of what to do about it and our commitment to treat both problems is emerging and skills are developing. Therefore, this Special Edition attempts to show where we are as a profession while we also search out new areas of exploration and study. This multi-faceted issue of the *Alcoholism Treatment Quarterly* will hopefully stimulate further research, offer information and guidelines for treatment and training, and encourage both the sexology and alcoholism fields to have further cooperation and joint ventures.

David J. Powell, Ph.D.

Alcohol
and Human Sexual Response

Sandra R. Leiblum, Ph.D.
Raymond C. Rosen, Ph.D.

Traditionally, alcohol has been widely regarded as a powerful facilitator, promoter, disinhibitor, and common accompaniment to sexual behavior of all types. In this context, alcohol remains a standard remedy for the sexually inhibited and inept, as well as enjoying a reputation for aphrodisiacal qualities among both users and abusers. However, along with its reputed powers as a sexual enhancer, alcohol has also been regarded by some as potentially destructive and detrimental to sexual responsivity when taken in excess. This review is intended to consider these two opposing views of alcohol's effects on sexual response in the light of current research.

Due to the influence of popular literature and conventional wisdom, there exists a well-known mythology concerning alcohol and sex. For example, two very commonly cited quotations in this regard are Ogden Nash's limerick: "Candy is dandy, But liquor is quicker" and Shakespeare's lines from the porter's speech in Macbeth: "It [alcohol] provokes and unprovokes: It provokes the desire, but it takes away the performance". Nevertheless, it is noteworthy that only in the last decade has there been a serious scientific effort to unravel the precise relationship between alcohol and sex.

In fact, what at first appeared to be a straightforward research question has turned out to be a complex and challenging experimental task. The question of how alcohol affects sexual response can be broken down in numerous ways. For instance, it is necessary to separate chronic from acute effects of alcohol consumption, the effects of varying dosage levels across different subject groups, and the relative contributions of pharmacological vs. psychological effects. Moreover, there have been some notable inconsistencies in the findings of various investigators attempting to replicate some basic studies. In addition, as noted by Carpenter and Armenti (1971), sexual

behavior is multifaceted and mediated by a variety of psychoneuro-
logical and hormonal mechanisms, and hence may be influenced by
alcohol in complex and nonlinear ways. Finally, Wilson (1981) has
recently concluded on the basis of a comprehensive review of the
literature that "the pharmacological effect of alcohol is confounded
with sexual opportunity . . . . (and) that the circumstances under
which it is consumed is the more important determinant of sexual
behavior" (p.35).

Along with the recent upsurge in scientific studies on alcohol and
sex, clinical concern regarding alcohol abuse and its effects on sexual behavior has markedly increased (Forrest, 1983). Sexual dysfunction among both male and female alcoholics is now commonly
acknowledged as a major clinical problem. In this regard, both the
short-term and long-term effects of alcohol are sources of concern to
the clinician, as well as alcohol's potential role in eliciting instances
of sexual aggression.

ACUTE EFFECTS OF ALCOHOL ON SEXUAL RESPONSE

Studies Involving Male Subjects

Early laboratory studies on alcohol and sex were primarily conducted using the prototypical male college student subjects. The use
of male subjects reflected in part the earlier availability of measurement technology (i.e., the penile plethysmograph), as well as the
not atypical bias of viewing males as the primary users and abusers
of alcohol. Nonetheless, in the past five years a number of studies
involving female subjects have been conducted and these will be reviewed in the following section.

The first study to directly assess the acute effects of alcohol consumption on male sexual response was carried out by Farkas and
Rosen (1976). These investigators administered four carefully controlled combinations of ethanol alcohol and orange juice to male
college students. When subjects reached the predetermined dosage
levels (0, 0.025, 0.050, and 0.075% Blood Alcohol Concentration),
penile tumescence was measured in response to the presentation of
an erotic movie. Regarding the pharmacological effects of alcohol
dosage levels on arousal, the results indicated that although there
was a slight increase in responsivity at the lowest BAC, it was followed by a significant and much greater decrease in arousal at the

higher dosage levels. Subjects' self report in this study corre-
sponded closely with the physiological results; the greatest subjective estimates of arousal occurred at the lowest alcohol dosage level.

Similar results were obtained in a study by Rubin and Henson
(1976) using comparable alcohol dosages (0.5, 1.0, and 1.5 ml/kg).
In this study sixteen volunteer male subjects again viewed erotic
stimuli in the laboratory while their penile tumescence responses
were recorded at each of the three different blood alcohol levels. A
repeated measures design was used, and the researchers also tested
the subjects ability to voluntarily control tumescence under both alcohol and placebo conditions. As in the Farkas and Rosen (1976)
study, Rubin and Henson found that moderate amounts of alcohol
were associated with some impairment of erectile response, whereas
at the highest alcohol dose major suppression of tumescence
occurred. Regarding the subjects' ability to voluntarily control erection, there was little evidence for alcohol's effects on facilitation or
suppression of response.

It is noteworthy that in both of the above studies alcohol did not
completely eliminate arousal even at the highest dosage levels.
While there was a significant response decrement in both studies, no
attempt was made to evaluate the subjects' ability to accomplish
intromission—perhaps the most crucial of "real-life" tests! An additional finding in the Rubin and Henson (1976) study was that most
of the subjects believed that alcohol enhanced sexual performance,
and this belief was unaffected by the subjects' laboratory experiences to the contrary.

A third study published in the same year (Briddell and Wilson,
1976) used a different methodological approach for assessing the
acute effects of alcohol on male sexual arousal. Forty-eight student
volunteers were randomly assigned to one of eight groups. Half of
the groups were told that alcohol would facilitate their sexual
arousal, while the other groups were told to expect a negative effect.
In addition, each of the groups received one of four alcohol dosages
(0.08, 0.5, 0.8, and 1.2 gms/kg). Arousal was again assessed by
measurement of penile tumescence in response to erotic stimuli. Results showed that arousal was inversely proportional to the amount
of alcohol consumed, and that this effect was uninfluenced by the
subjects' expectations.

However, when Wilson and Lawson (1976) subsequently manip-
ulated the subjects' belief that they had consumed either alcohol or
placebo, those subjects who believed they had ingested alcohol

showed increased tumescence compared to those who believed they had drunk only tonic water. Interestingly, no main effect of alcohol was found in this study, apparently due to the fact that only small amounts of alcohol were given (0.5-0.6 gms/kg).

In the most recent, and perhaps most provocative study to date conducted by Wilson and his colleagues (Wilson, Niaura, and Adler, in press), an attempt was made to assess the effects of alcohol ingestion on the cognitive processing of sexual stimuli. This study was designed to serve as a laboratory analogue for alcohol's effects on performance anxiety and the consequent effects on penile tumescence in male social drinkers. Using a similar balanced placebo design as in the above study (Wilson and Lawson, 1976), subjects again received either alcohol or placebo, and were required to perform either a simple or complex cognitive task while listening to erotic tapes. The cognitive tasks consisted of copying a list of random digits (simple task), or classifying a list of random digits (complex task).

While it is beyond the scope of this paper to review the intricacies of all the findings from this study, several results deserve mention. In the condition of the simple cognitive task, the belief that the subjects had consumed alcohol enhanced arousal as in the Wilson and Lawson (1976) study. On the other hand, the pharmacological effect of alcohol was manifested only in the condition of the complex cognitive task, i.e., alcohol ingestion produced decreased arousal when subjects were required to process complex stimuli. These findings are perhaps due to the different attentional demands of the two cognitive tasks and the differential effects of alcohol or the expectation of alcohol on each. The real-life implication of these findings is that alcohol's effects on sexual performance are likely to vary depending upon the degree of comfort the male feels in the sexual situation. Under conditions of low stress (e.g., simple cognitive tasks), sexual arousal may be enhanced by the expectation of alcohol. On the other hand, under conditions of high stress, (e.g., complex cognitive tasks), performance will be diminished by the pharmacological effects of alcohol.

However, not all researchers in this area agree that the primary pharmacological effect of alcohol is to diminish arousal. For example, Langevin et al. (1983) recently studied the effects of three different alcohol dosage levels (0.0, 0.5, and 1.0 BAL) on tumescence responses to erotic slides of varying content categories. The subjects for this study were forty-eight paid, male volunteers without any history of alcohol abuse. Unlike the other studies reported above, these researchers found that alcohol, even at the highest dosage level, did not significantly reduce the overall level of erection responses achieved. This apparently inconsistent result may have been due to a number of key methodological differences in this study. A volumetric method of penile measurement was used instead of the more typical circumference technique, a wide range of erotic slides was presented in an unusual order and sequence, and subjects were tested early in the morning as opposed to the more usual afternoon or evening times. Finally, as Langevin et al. point out, none of the above studies have controlled carefully for the prior drinking histories or other potentially confounding characteristics of the subjects, which may also account for some of the differences found.

Thus far only one study to date has examined the acute effects of alcohol on the male orgasmic/ejaculatory response (Malatesta et al., 1979). For purposes of this study, twenty-four male volunteers ("social drinkers"), were observed during masturbation to orgasm in the laboratory. Subjects were brought to one of four blood alcohol levels (0.0%, 0.03%, 0.06%, and 0.09%) as latency to ejaculation was measured. Results clearly indicated a marked impairment of ejaculation at the higher alcohol dosage levels, as ten of the subjects were completely unable to ejaculate at the 0.09% level. Also significant were the subjective responses of the subjects which similarly showed decreased pleasurability and intensity of orgasm at the higher alcohol dosage levels. The authors also point out, however, that the moderate increase in latency of ejaculation at the lower alcohol dosage levels may serve an adaptive function in prolonging intercourse in certain situations.

On balance the above studies suggest independent and interactive effects of the pharmacological and psychosocial determinants mediating the influence of alcohol on sexual response. Pharmacologically, alcohol appears to impair male sexual arousal and orgasm at the higher blood alcohol levels. Sexual desire, however, is influenced greatly by the setting and circumstances under which alcohol is consumed (Wilson, 1981).

Studies Involving Female Subjects

Laboratory investigation of acute alcohol effects in women only began after the development of the vaginal photoplethysmograph (Sintchak and Geer, 1975), an instrument for measuring vaginal blood flow and thereby sexual arousal. Using this device, Wilson and Lawson (1976) tested the effects of four alcohol doses (0.05, 0.25, 0.50, and 0.75) on sixteen female social drinkers. All subjects were shown an erotic film and vaginal blood flow responses as well as subjective reports of arousal at each dosage level were recorded.

While the pharmacological effects of alcohol on vaginal blood flow appeared to mirror the negative results found with male tumescence, the self-reports of the female subjects produced some unexpected findings. Firstly, women predicted that they would experience more arousal at higher alcohol levels. Indeed, despite the impaired vaginal blood flow responses at the higher blood alcohol levels, the women reported feeling more aroused. The authors have interpreted this finding as perhaps due to women's inaccuracy in identifying and labeling physiological cues of sexual arousal.

This finding was replicated in a second study by Wilson and Lawson (1978) in which the same balanced placebo design previously used with male subjects was employed with female social drinkers. Again, the authors found that even a moderate alcohol dose (0.4 g/kg.) depressed vaginal blood flow significantly. On the other hand, subjective reports of arousal increased under both conditions of alcohol intake or the belief that alcohol was consumed.

Regarding the effects of alcohol intoxication on orgasmic response in women, Malatesta et al. (1982) evaluated the effects of four blood alcohol concentrations (0.0, 0.025, 0.050, 0.075) on latency and intensity of orgasm during masturbation in eighteen university women. As in the Wilson and Lawson studies, vaginal photoplethysmograph results indicated a progressive impairment of physiological responding with increased intoxication. Orgasmic latency clearly increased, while the intensity of orgasm appeared to be diminished. Paradoxically, subjects reported higher levels of subjective arousal and orgasmic pleasurability at the moderate and high alcohol dosage levels.

Taken together, these three studies suggest that alcohol seems to significantly depress physiological arousal in women, while nevertheless permitting the belief that alcohol facilitates sexual enjoyment. Overall, there appear to be major similarities in the acute effects of alcohol on sexual response in male and female social drinkers, with the exception of the findings of Wilson and Lawson discussed above. Essentially, it appears that attributions of sexual arousal under conditions of alcohol intoxication (real or imagined) are maintained for women, despite physiological evidence to the contrary. Males, on the other hand, appear more likely to modify their attribution of arousal depending upon their awareness of physiological arousal.

CHRONIC EFFECTS OF ALCOHOL ON SEXUAL FUNCTION IN MALES AND FEMALES

Shifting focus to the long-term effects of alcohol abuse on sexual function, one finds a number of problems parallel to those identified in the preceding section. Specifically, the extent and chronicity of abuse is quite variable from one subject to another and is not always adequately controlled for in clinical studies. In addition, the pre-alcoholic sexual competency of the individual is typically not assessed, and hence, there may be some confounding between subject variables and long-term effects. In fact, the impact of alcohol on sexual function may vary considerably depending upon the particular stage of the individual's alcoholic career. For example, Forrest (1983) notes that early in the male alcoholic's career a few drinks may serve to disinhibit and facilitate greater sexual initiative, especially on the part of sexually inept males. Similarly, Forrest also notes that female drinkers may initially experience more confidence in their femininity and sexual attractiveness when drinking.

Other problems also exist in identifying the causal mechanisms involved in sexual impairment of the chronic alcoholic. Explanations to date have focused on underlying endocrine, neurological, psychological, and interpersonal disturbances that may all result from long-term alcohol abuse. Wilsnack (1980) summarizes six possible physiological mechanisms which might account for the disruptive effects of chronic alcoholism on sexual function. Specifically, these include the acute depressant effects of alcohol on sexual response, the disruption of gonadal hormone metabolism as a result of liver damage, reduced sexual sensation due to alcohol induced neuropathy, organic brain damage causing impairment of both interpersonal and sexual interest, and various medical problems associated with alcoholism (e.g., diabetes, hypertension) that might, in turn, lead to sexual problems. Indeed, in the most severe cases of alcohol abuse, major deterioration occurs in all aspects of the biopsychosocial system. This general deterioration effect makes it difficult, if not impossible, to parcel out specific etiological mechanisms in individual cases.

Studies of Male Alcoholics

All aspects of the male sexual response cycle may be negatively affected by chronic alcohol abuse (Mandell and Miller, 1983; Forrest, 1983). However, there appears to be accumulating evidence that the arousal phase of the response cycle, and the erectile response in particular, is most dramatically impaired.

Past studies of impotence associated with alcoholism have reported an incidence range of 8% (Lemere and Smith, 1973) to 54% (Whalley, 1978). More recently, Mandell and Miller (1983) have reported on the results of an in-depth interview with forty-four male alcoholics admitted to an out-patient treatment program. The authors observed that frequency, duration and quantity of drinking were proportionately related to sexual impairment. Specifically, it was found that during periods of heavy drinking 59% of the male patients had experienced erectile dysfunction, while 48% reported ejaculatory difficulties. Overall, 84% of the patients had experienced some kind of sexual difficulty in association with alcohol abuse.

An obvious methodological criticism of the above studies is the reliance on the self-report of the respondents and the absence of objective assessment of sexual dysfunction. A notable exception is a recent study by Snyder and Karacan (1981) which assessed nocturnal penile tumescence (NPT) responses in a sample of twenty-six chronic male alcoholics in the process of detoxification. NPT is a widely used method of differentiating organic from psychogenic impotence by means of sleep laboratory monitoring of nocturnal erections (Rosen, 1983). Snyder and Karacan found a number of significant differences in the erectile function of their chronic alcoholic group as compared to an age-matched non-alcoholic control group.

The alcoholic subjects displayed reduced latency to tumescence (slower erections), decreased number and rigidity of erections, and more semi-erections than the control subjects. This finding indicates that the sexual difficulties associated with chronic alcohol abuse are due, in part, to organic factors, probably of neurological origin. Although the subjects in this study were only three weeks into a detoxification program, the magnitude and extent of the erectile impairment suggests the likelihood of irreversible damage.

Jensen (1979) has reported that erectile dysfunction in alcoholic men is significantly related to both age and marital status. In this study, men over forty and single alcoholic men were more likely to report impotence, although the duration of the alcoholism was not significantly related to sexual dysfunction. Another finding in this study was that 80% of the alcoholics reported that their partners were sexually disinterested when they were drunk. Thus, the social rejection and lack of arousability of the alcoholic's partner may mediate some part of his resulting dysfunction.

Other authors have also emphasized the disruptive effects of chronic alcoholism on sexual and interpersonal relationships. For example, Kolodny, Masters, and Johnson (1979) have described a typical interactional pattern in which the wife of the alcoholic withdraws from sexual activity as a form of retaliation for her husband's undesirable (drinking) behavior. This, in turn, often leads to coercive or abusive behavior on the part of the intoxicated husband, and increasing hostility and withdrawal on the part of the wife. These authors have also emphasized the sexual and interpersonal difficulties of the alcoholic in recovery. Depression and poor self-esteem are common in the early stages of rehabilitation, and may lead to further sexual difficulties.

On a more positive note, Forrest (1983) has recently described a range of treatment options for overcoming sexual dysfunction in male alcoholics. Beginning with an emphasis on the need for sobriety during treatment, Forrest recommends a complete medical and psychological evaluation prior to initiating therapy. In cases where there does not appear to be organic impairment, conventional sex therapy procedures may be instituted, with special attention being paid to the issues of resentment and anger in the relationship. For this reason, marital or couples counselling is typically viewed as an integral part of the therapy. In following this general approach, Forrest reports a success rate of approximately 70% in male alcoholics entering therapy and remaining sober for at least one year. These reportedly high success rates may be unduly optimistic, and remain to be substantiated by other investigators.

The Alcohol Feminization Syndrome

A particular syndrome associated with advanced alcoholic liver disease is the feminization syndrome observed in some male alcoholics (Van Thiel, 1980; Chiao & Van Thiel, 1983). Clinical observations of men with this problem have shown impotence, testicular atrophy, and gynecomastia in varying degrees. According to Van Thiel and Lester (1977), two interrelated processes are responsible for these effects: hypoandrogenization, a pathological decline in androgen production, which results in diminished circulating testosterone levels; and hyperestrogenization, or excessive levels of plasma estrone, estradiol, and prolactin, resulting in varying degrees of feminization.

Recent research on this syndrome has tended to focus on Leydig cell failure in chronic alcoholic men as a possible important mediating factor (Chiao & Van Thiel, 1983). At present there are, however, a number of unresolved neuroendocrine issues in understanding this syndrome. For example, whether the feminization process is triggered by a central disturbance in the hypothalamic-pituitary axis or is attributable to peripheral changes associated with liver damage remains to be investigated.

Studies of Female Alcoholics

Recognition of sexual difficulties in the female alcoholic is a relatively recent phenomenon. In their review of the literature up to that time, Carpenter and Armenti (1971) remarked that "Most experts comment on human sexual behavior and alcohol as though only males drink and have sexual interests" (p. 521). Clearly, however, the problems of female alcoholics ought to be given equal consideration, as recent studies have indicated that chronic alcohol abuse can be as deleterious for the female alcoholic as her male counterpart.

Just as for the male, the female alcoholic typically progresses through a series of stages of physical and psychological deterioration which negatively impact on sexual function. In the early stages alcohol may serve a disinhibiting function in overcoming high levels of sexual guilt and low self-control. Pinhas (1980) tested this hypothesis by administering two psychological inventories which assessed sex guilt and perceived locus of control to thirty-four recovering alcoholic women. Results showed that these women had significantly higher ratings of sex guilt and lower perceived self-control as compared with a matched control group. Pinhas (1980) suggests that alcohol, either because of its pharmacological or expectancy effects, permits alcoholic women to overcome their sexual inhibitions and feelings of personal inadequacy and overlook the negative effect of being regarded as a female alcoholic.

Several other recent studies of recovering female alcoholics have produced a range of findings regarding alcohol abuse and female sexuality. Covington (1983) compared thirty-five women in an alcohol recovery program to appropriate controls and found a significantly higher rate of sexual dysfunction in the alcoholic women. Specifically, 64% of the alcoholic women indicated a lack of sexual interest, 61% a lack of sexual arousal, and 64% complained of the absence of orgasm. This author also reported a high association between drinking and sexual activity prior to sobriety. She notes that "the major love relationship in an alcoholic's life is with the liquor bottle." The same paradoxical finding that was noted earlier in regard to the acute effects of alcohol on female sexual response is also evident in Covington's work on chronic female abusers. The alcoholic women believed that alcohol contributes positively to sexual experience, while their own clinical histories indicate the reverse.

Apter-Marsh (1983) obtained similar findings in an interview study with sixty-one heterosexual, middle-class recovering alcoholic women. This author again found a similar pattern of arousal and orgasmic dysfunction during periods of alcohol abuse. Of particular interest, however, was Apter-Marsh's finding that women reported different sexual concerns during periods of active drinking and later sobriety. During the drinking years, major concerns expressed by the respondents were promiscuity, guilt, shame, deception, pregnancy fears and general sexual inhibition. During sobriety, on the other hand, concerns focused on relationship and intimacy issues such as fears of commitment, partner unavailability, and communication difficulties, in addition to continuing sexual inhibition.

An important finding reported by several independent investigators is the high prevalence of sexual and aggressive victimization in the clinical histories of alcoholic women. For example, Murphy, Coleman, Hoon, and Scott (1980) found that half of the seventy-four alcoholic women in their study reported being the victim of rape, either as a child or adult. Similarly, Covington (1983) found that 34% of her alcoholic subjects were victims of either incest or rape, as contrasted with less than half this number in the control sample. While the reasons for this disturbingly high incidence of sexual victimization in alcoholic women need further study, certain clinical implications can be drawn. Specifically, such abuse may lead to a heightened sense of interpersonal distrust and sexual discomfort in adult sexual relationships, thereby increasing the woman's vulnerability to the perceived disinhibiting effects of alcohol. Further, sexual orientation may be affected as a result of a generalized distrust of men. In this regard, Wilsnack (1976) suggests that alcoholic women are insecure about their femininity and have homosexual conflicts which they attempt to suppress via alcohol.

Taken together, the above studies suggest that women view alcohol as facilitating sexual response, and alcoholic women in particular, tend to engage in sex when under the influence of alcohol. Under these conditions they believe that alcohol permits disinhibition of performance anxiety and personal feelings of sexual inadequacy. When sober, however, they acknowledge that alcohol retards orgasmic responsivity and serves as a means of avoidance of more serious concerns about sexual adequacy, intimacy, and interpersonal relationships.

ALCOHOL AND SEXUAL AGGRESSION

A final area of research that warrants attention is the oft-cited association between alcohol abuse and acts of sexual aggression. Although a complete review of the extensive literature on this topic is beyond the scope of the present paper, a few salient points are worth noting here. A number of investigators have found a significant correlation between alcohol intoxication and sexually aggressive behavior (Gebhard et al., 1965; Amir, 1967; Rada, 1974, 1975). For example, in an investigation of a large sample of committed rapists (Rada, 1974), 50% reported being intoxicated at the time of the assault. Further, 35% of these rapists were diagnosed as alcoholic by the research team.

While this prevalence rate is typical of a number of studies showing a relatively high association between alcoholism and sexual misconduct, the causal relationships involved remain to be articulated. For example, the degree of alcohol consumption at the time of the offense, a key factor in the presumed chain of events, may be highly variable and is typically only inferred from the retrospective self-reports of the offenders (Wilson, 1981). Further, the category of sexual offenders includes a variety of sub-types (i.e., rapists, pedophiles, incest offenders), and the motivational and personality characteristics of these subgroups have been shown to vary considerably. Thus, the role of alcohol as a disinhibitor/facilitator of sexual misconduct might differ across studies. Finally, Wilson (1981) also notes that offenders may exaggerate their degree of intoxication as a form of legal defense, further biasing the self-report data on which the association is based.

One of the more provocative questions in this area has been raised by Langevin and his associates (in press). Specifically, Langevin poses the question of how it is that alcohol is supposed to both suppress sexual function at high dosages, as well as permitting some men to perform sexually in instances of sexual aggression. After reviewing the available literature on this topic, Langevin raises a number of hypotheses as follows. Firstly, it is possible that the studies reviewed above on the acute effects of alcohol ingestion on sexual arousal may have unduly emphasized the suppressive effects, particularly if one assumes that certain individuals can develop tolerance to prolonged drinking. Also, this author notes that several studies have indicated elevated plasma testosterone levels in some violent offenders, and that high testosterone levels may be positively correlated with both aggressiveness and enhanced sexual arousability. Therefore, the use of alcohol by such individuals may not dampen sexual arousal sufficiently in view of the overriding impact of higher androgen levels.

Clearly, the relationship between alcohol and sexual aggression is much in need of further study. One recent line of research that complicates the issue even further concerns the effects of alcohol, or the expectation of alcohol consumption, on elicitation of arousal to deviant stimuli in non-offender, non-alcoholic subjects. For example, Briddell et al. (1978) used the balanced placebo design to assess tumescence responses to coercive and non-coercive sexual stimuli in male social drinkers. Results indicated that subjects who believed that they had consumed alcohol showed greater erection responses to the deviant stimuli than subjects who believed that they had received the placebo dose. On the other hand, the pharmacological effect of alcohol was not significant in this study.

More recently, Langevin et al. (in press) have found that in a similar sample alcohol consumption led to more indiscriminate arousal to a wide range of erotic stimuli, i.e., at moderate or high alcohol dosages, subjects were more arousable by both mild and atypical sexual stimuli. The implication from both of these studies is that alcohol may act, even in non-offender males, as a cue for sexual misconduct. However, it is unclear at present whether this effect is primarily due to pharmacological factors or the social disinhibition effects of alcohol.

One can anticipate an increasing social and scientific emphasis on research into alcohol's role in sexual disinhibition and aggression in the years to come. As societal awareness is focused on the distressingly high prevalence of rape, incest, child sexual abuse and other sexual crimes, and as the association of alcohol intoxication with these offenses is documented, it is crucial to determine the causative determinants of this association.

CONCLUSION

A number of issues have been highlighted in this review. Firstly, the effects of alcohol on sexual function need to be considered from both the perspective of acute and chronic consumption. Short-term alcohol effects, which have been investigated primarily in social drinker subjects, have been shown to be influenced by both pharmacological and attitudinal factors. Male and female differences in this regard are especially interesting, and have been discussed at some length. On the other hand, studies of chronic alcohol abuse have yielded a consistent picture of sexual and interpersonal deterioration in most cases. The possible causative factors in this regard are multiple and overlapping.

Several important methodological concerns have also been raised in this review. Unfortunately, much of the clinical literature on sexual dysfunction associated with alcoholism has been based on retrospective and subjective self-report data. Furthermore, the definitions of alcohol abuse and sexual disturbance have varied greatly from one study to another. Studies of alcoholic subjects are typically conducted during the early stages of the recovery period, and it is unclear to what extent this has affected the findings reported. Clearly, there is a major need for more long-term prospective research if the issues are to be adequately addressed.

REFERENCES

Amir, M. Alcohol and forcible rape. *British Journal of Addiction*, 1967, *62*, 219-232.

Apter-Marsh, M. The sexual behavior of alcoholic women while drinking and during sobriety. Paper presented at the 6th World Congress of Sexology, Washington, D.C., May, 1983.

Briddell, D. W., & Wilson, G. T. The effects of alcohol and expectancy set on male sexual arousal. *Journal of Abnormal Psychology*, 1976, *85*, 225-234.

Briddell, D. W., Rimm, D. C., Caddy, G. R., Krawitz, G., Sholis, D., & Wunderlin, R. J. Effects of alcohol on cognitive set on sexual arousal to deviant stimuli. *Journal of Abnormal Psychology*, 1978, *87*, 418-430.

Carpenter, A. & Armenti, N. P. Some effects of ethanol on human sexual and aggressive behavior. In B. Kissen & H. Begleiter (Eds.), *The Biology of Alcoholism*. New York: Plenum, 1971.

Chiao, Y. & Van Thiel, D. H. Biochemical mechanisms that contribute to alcohol-induced hypogonadism in the male. *Alcoholism: Clinical and Experimental Research*, 1983, *7*, 131-134.

Covington, S. Sex and alcohol: What do women tell us. Paper presented at the 6th World Congress of Sexology, Washington, D.C., May, 1983.

Farkas, G. & Rosen, R. C. The effects of ethanol on male sexual arousal. *Journal of Alcohol Studies*, 1976, *37*, 265-272.

Forrest, G. G. *Alcoholism and human sexuality*. Springfield, Ill.: Charles C. Thomas, 1983.

Gebhard, P. H., Gagnon, J. H., Pomeroy, W. B., & Christenson, C. V. *Sex offenders*. New York: Harper and Row, 1965.

Jensen, S. B. Sexual customs and sexual dysfunction in alcoholics. *British Journal of Sexual Medicine*, 1979, *54*, 30-34.

Kolodny, R. C., Masters, W. H., & Johnson, V. E. *Textbook of sexual medicine*. Boston: Little Brown, 1979.

Langevin, R., Bain, J., Ben-Aron, M., & Coulthard, R. Sexual aggression: Constructing a predictive equation. In R. Langevin (Ed.) *Erotic preference, gender identity, and aggression in men* (in press).

Langevin, R., Ben-Aron, M., Coulthard, R., & Day, D. The effect of alcohol on penile erection. In R. Langevin (Ed.), *Erotic preference, gender identity, and aggression in men*, (in press).

Lemere, F. & Smith, J. W. Alcohol-induced sexual impotence. *American Journal of Psychiatry*, 1973, *130*, 212-213.

Mandell, W., & Miller, C. M. Male sexual dysfunction as related to alcohol consumption: A pilot study. *Alcoholism: Clinical and Experimental Research*, 1983, *7*, 65-69.

Malatesta, V. J., Pollack, R. H., Wilbanks, W. A., & Adams, H. E. Alcohol effects on the orgasmic-ejaculatory response in human males. *Journal of Sex Research*, 1979, *15*, 101-107.

Malatesta, V. J., Pollack, R. H., Crotty, T. D., & Peacock, L. J. Acute alcohol intoxication and female orgasmic response. *Journal of Sex Research*, 1982, *18*, 1-17.

Murphy, W. D., Coleman, E., Hoon, E., & Scott, C. Sexual dysfunction and treatment in alcoholic women. *Sexuality and Disability*, 1980, *3*, 240-255.

Pinhas, V. Sex guilt and sexual control in women alcoholics in early sobriety. *Sexuality and Disability*, 1980, *3*, 256-269.

Rada, R. T. Alcoholism and forcible rape. *American Journal of Psychiatry*, 1973, *132*, 444-446.

Rada, R. T. Alcohol and rape. *Medical Aspects of Human Sexuality*, 1975, *9*, 48-65.

Rosen, R. C. Clinical issues in the assessment and treatment of impotence. *Behavior Therapist*, 1983.

Rubin, H. B., & Henson, D. E. Effects of alcohol on male sexual responding. *Psychopharmacology*, 1976, *47*, 123-134.

Sintchak, G., & Geer, J. A vaginal plethysmograph system. *Psychophysiology*, 1975, *12*, 113-115.

Snyder, S., & Karacan, I. Effects of chronic alcoholism on nocturnal penile tumescence. *Psychosomatic Medicine*. 1981, *43*, 423-429.

Van Thiel, D. H., & Lester, R. Alcoholism: Its effect on hypothalamic pituitary gonadal function. *Gastroentorology*, 1976, *71*, 318-327.

Van Thiel, D. H. Alcohol and its effect on endocrine functioning. *Alcoholism: Clinical and Experimental Research*, 1980, *4*, 44-49.

Whalley, L. J. Sexual adjustment of male alcoholics. *Acta Psychiatrica Scandinavia*, 1978, *58*, 281-298.

Wilsnack, S. C. Alcohol, sexuality, and reproductive dysfunction in women. In E. L. Abel (Ed.), *Fetal alcohol syndrome: Vol. II. Human studies*. Boca Raton, Fla.: CRC Press, 1980.

Wilson, G. T., The effects of alcohol on human sexual behavior *Advances in Substance Abuse*, 1981, *2*, 1-40.

Wilson, G. T., & Lawson, D. M. Expectancies, alcohol and sexual arousal in male social drinkers. *Journal of Abnormal Psychology*, 1976 (a), *85*, 587-594.

Wilson, G. T., & Lawson, D. M. Expectancies, alcohol, and sexual arousal in women. *Journal of Abnormal Psychology*, 1978, *87*, 358-367.

Wilson, G. T. Niaura, R., & Adler, J. Affect, alcohol, and selective attention.

Socio-Sexual Issues
in the Using and Recovering Alcoholic

David Smith, M.D.
Mildred Apter-Marsh, Ph.D.
John Buffum, Pharm.D.
Charles Moser, Ph.D.
Don Wesson, M.D.

The disease of alcoholism is the third leading killer in the United States and represents one of our country's major health problems. Over 13 million individuals in the United States are alcoholics, representing approximately 7% of the adult population. It has been estimated that alcoholism costs the country over 40·billion dollars in terms of health care costs, lost productivity, accidents, crime, and is a major contributor to over half the fatal auto accidents in the United States. Each year, approximately 25,000 individuals die and 1.5 million people are injured by drunk drivers. To be more specific, over 60% of the homicides involve alcohol in both the offender and victim. Sixty-five percent of aggressive sexual acts against children and 39% of aggressive sexual acts against women involve alcohol by the offender. Alcohol abuse also represents the number one substance abuse problem in adolescents. Over 85% of all 10th to 12th graders have at some time or another consumed the psychoactive drug, alcohol. Fifteen percent of 10th to 12th graders report heavy drinking, and in high school students 36% of the regular drinkers have had two or more accidental injuries serious enough to interfere with their daily activities. Auto accidents and suicides are two of the leading causes of death in the adolescent population, and both are deeply involved with alcohol and other psychoactive drugs.

Alcohol abuse has been growing steadily among adolescents and is by far the most commonly used drug in this population. The health care system is greatly affected by the problem of alcoholism; 10% of the adults entering a private physician's office are alcoholics, with 15% to 40% of adult admissions to general hospitals being due to alcohol related problems. The children of using alcoholics are also adversely affected. They have a wide range of problems from fetal alcohol syndrome to being at a high risk for hyperactivity, emotional problems and child abuse. There is an evolving awareness that alcoholism is a primary disease with its causative factors being an interplay of both genetics and environment. It is a multifactorial illness that may involve either episodic or daily increasing abuse of alcohol, with either pattern producing physical dependency with a number of important biomedical, psychological and social sequelae ranging from cirrhosis of the liver, depression, behavioral problems such as marital difficulties and loss of job.

Given the complicated nature of the disease of alcoholism in our society, there have been attempts to be precise in the diagnostic criteria for alcoholism. The DSM III describes two different patterns of alcoholism (the dysfunctional use of alcohol); alcohol abuse and alcohol dependence. Alcohol abuse is characterized by:

1. A pattern of pathological alcohol use such as a need for daily drink to the presence of binges or blackouts;
2. Impairment in social or occupational functioning due to alcohol use such as loss of job or legal difficulties, and;
3. Duration of alcohol disturbance of at least one month.

Alcohol dependence is characterized by two major criteria:

1. Either a pattern of pathological alcohol abuse or impairment in social or occupational functioning due to alcohol;
2. Evidence of physical dependence on alcohol with tolerance and withdrawal.

Tolerance is defined as the need to increase the dose of alcohol in order to achieve the desired effect with withdrawal having characteristic signs and symptoms including tremor, tachycardia, restlessness with the most extreme manifestations being alcohol withdrawal seizure and psychosis.

The direct toxic effects of alcohol in the body including the central nervous system are categorized in the DSM III under substance-induced organic mental disorders, and include alcohol intoxication, alcohol withdrawal, delirium tremens (DT's) and alcohol hallucinosis.

These DSM III criteria developed out of the psychiatric system which partially overlaps and sometimes conflicts diagnostically with terminology used by addictionologists, who define alcoholism as a disease (Smith,1984). Alcohol abuse is defined more as episodic dysfunctional use with alcoholism diagnosis in its early stages not requiring evidence of tissue dependence. The general formula for understanding the causation of any addictive disease including alcoholism is addictive disease = genetics + environment. In the disease concept of alcoholism, more emphasis is placed on the psychobiological predisposition. For example, with familial forms of alcoholism, blackouts are perceived as an early diagnostic sign of alcoholism, manifesting altered response to the drug early in the individual's drug taking career. Whereas other individuals who develop blackouts may represent a late stage of alcoholism as a consequence of the neurological damage induced by alcohol. Figure 1 illustrates the classic representation of the alcoholism cycle. Table 1 summarizes some of the physical, social and psychological dysfunctions produced by alcohol, one of which is sexual dysfunction.

The using alcoholic escalates his dosage as the disease progresses and may start manifesting ejaculatory and erectile failure in the male, desire phase disorder in the female. Alcohol induced sexual dysfunction as well as impairment in personal relationships can be a major negative consequence of alcoholism which may interact with other negative consequences. For example, blackouts, where the individual abuses alcohol and has retrograde amnesia. Losing memory while still retaining motor function is a frequent symptom seen in the alcoholic. Blackouts may last for minutes or days but usually occur over a several hour period and the frequency is associated with the severity and duration of alcoholism, although in certain individuals, the onset of blackouts may occur early in the individual's drinking career. Female alcoholics, for example, often become disinhibited when they drink in a social situation and end up with a strange man in a sexual setting they are not familiar with, wake up the next morning in bed with that man and have no recollection of how they got there. Such alcohol-induced blackouts in altered social-sexual response become a great issue of embarrassment, humiliation and guilt for the individual.

Heavy drinking in males is highest during ages 18 to 20, dips in the early 30's and then begins to increase to a second peak during the ages 35 to 39. In women, the highest proportion of heavy drinking occurs in ages 21 to 29, dips slightly in the early 30's and then levels off in the late 30's to early 40's. In studies of high school stu-

FIGURE I
A CONCEPTUAL MODEL OF ALCOHOLISM

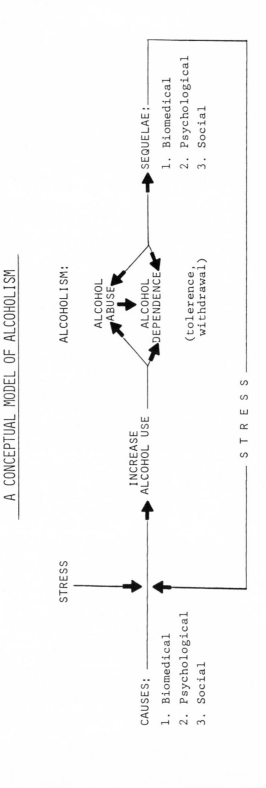

TABLE 1

PHYSICAL, PSYCHOLOGICAL AND SOCIAL DYSFUNCTION PRODUCED BY ALCOHOL

PHYSICAL	PSYCHOLOGICAL
Esophagitis	Loneliness
Esophageal Varices	Guilt
Gastritis	Dependency.
Pancreatitis	Denial
Fatty Liver	Craving for Alcohol
Hepatitis	Anxiety
Cirrhosis	Angry Outbursts
Portal Hypertension	Depression
Nutritional Deficiency, especially vitamins (thiamine, folate)	Suicidal Ideation
	Hallucinosis
Hypothyroidism	Paranoia
Sexual Dysfunction (impotence, amenorrhea)	Other Drug Use
Cardiomyopathy	SOCIAL
Hypertension	Family Problems (marital, child abuse)
Increased risk for Cancer (mouth, pharynx, larynx, esophagus, liver, pancreas)	Inadequate Shelter
	Financial Problems
Pneumonia	Vocational Problems
Tuberculosis	Automobile Accidents
Myopathy	Legal Problems
Peripheral Neuropathy	Social Isolation
Fractures	
Subdural Hematoma	
Seizures	
Intoxication	
Blackouts	
Delirium Tremens	
Cerebellar Degeneration	
Werknicke-Korsakoff Syndrome	
Dementia	
Birth Defects (fetal alcohol syndrome)	

dents, 30% to 60% use alcohol at least once per month and 1% to 3% report daily use. Adler and Kindle (1981) found evidence to support the notion of a developmental sequence of substance abuse in adolescents where the abuse of alcohol was correlated to the abuse of other drugs. It is apparent that alcohol abuse alone and in combination with other substances occurs during the age group in which psycho-sexual patterns are developing, or when the individual may be potentially at their peak level of sexuality and reproductive capacity. The latter issue becomes particularly important in the female if the woman drinks heavily during pregnancy. There is a high incidence of alcohol-induced fetal alcohol syndrome in children born to these mothers. Although alcoholism and alcohol-prescription drug dependence is a significant problem in the elderly, there is a general drop in the rate of heavy drinking in both sexes in the early 50's and 60's. This is in part due to financial limitations and the early death rate of alcoholics.

Approximately 10% to 15% of diagnosed alcoholics may have a major psychiatric illness including thought disorder, major depression or bi-polar affective disorder. This underlying psychopathology may itself produce impairment of sexual functioning such as desire phase disorders associated with depression. However in many active alcoholics, depression and other psychological symptoms are more a consequence of drinking, and will disappear when the individual goes into abstinence.

Alcoholism is a multifactorial illness with multiple causes complicating factors. However, once the diagnosis of alcoholism is made, it is important to define a treatment sequence based on the point of entry of the individual into the treatment system, and to determine what elements of the treatment plan can be implemented at what stage of the individual's recovery.

Kanas has defined four phases in the treatment plan for the alcoholic (Tables 2 - 5). Phase 1 deals with the acute crisis, whether it is an alcohol overdose that can be life-threatening, or an acute medical crisis or severe withdrawal that involves detoxification for the alcohol-dependent individual to be safely withdrawn from the drug. This may be much less of an issue with the episodic alcohol abuser;

TABLE 2
TREATMENT ISSUES IN ALCOHOLISM
Phase One: Acute Crisis

TREATMENT DIMENSION	TYPICAL PROBLEMS	POSSIBLE SOLUTIONS
Biomedical	GI Bleeding, Pneumonia, Delirium Tremens	Hospitalization Appropriate Medical Intervention
Psychological	Hallucinosis, Paranoia, Suicidal Ideation	Hospitalization Appropriate Psychiatric Intervention
Social	Family Violence	Hospitalization Appropriate Psychiatric Intervention Family Therapy Home Visit

TABLE 3

TREATMENT ISSUES IN ALCOHOLISM
Phase Two: Withdrawal from Alcohol

TREATMENT DIMENSION	TYPICAL PROBLEMS	POSSIBLE SOLUTIONS
Biomedical	Impending DTs, Withdrawal Effects, Acute Medical Problems	Medical or Social Model Detoxification Outpatient Detoxification Appropriate Medical Intervention
Psychological	Denial, Worry about Health, Stressful Life Events	Counseling Brief Individual or Group Therapy
Social	Inadequate Shelter, Financial Problems	Counseling Social Services Referral

TABLE 4

TREATMENT ISSUES IN ALCOHOLISM
Phase Three: Sequelae of Alcoholism

TREATMENT DIMENSION	TYPICAL PROBLEMS	POSSIBLE SOLUTIONS
Biomedical	Chronic Medical Problems Malnutrition	Appropriate Medical Intervention Vitamin Supplements, Proper Diet, Exercise Disulfiram
Psychological	Denial, Depression, Guilt, Stressful Life Events, Psychological Craving	Counseling, Brief Individual or Group Therapy Antidepressants Lithium Carbonate Behavioral Techniques
Social	Family, Housing, Vocational, and Legal Problems Loneliness Unfilled Leisure Time	Counseling Social Services Referral Family Therapy Recreational Therapy Alcoholics Anonymous, Al-Anon, Alateen Alcoholic Halfway House

much more of an issue with the daily high dose alcoholic who may also be abusing other psychoactive drugs such as the benzodiazepines or barbiturates, which may complicate the dependency and withdrawal picture. After the acute medical crisis is dealt with, the detoxification plan is to be evaluated and implemented depending on the severity of the individual's dependence. Patients with a very high level of alcohol dependence and medical debilitation may suffer the life-threatening alcohol withdrawal delirium tremens and

TABLE 5
TREATMENT ISSUES IN ALCOHOLISM
Phase Four: Predisposing Causes

TREATMENT DIMENSION	TYPICAL PROBLEMS	POSSIBLE SOLUTIONS
Biomedical	Genetic Factors	Counseling
Psychological	Neurotic and Personality Disorders, Major Affective Disorders, Schizophrenia	Long-term Individual or Group Therapy Antidepressants Lithium Carbonate Major Tranquilizers
Social	Sociocultural and Familial Influences	Counseling

may require hospitalization, appropriate medication and medical management including careful monitoring of vital signs and IV fluids (with electrolytes and vitamins). With treatment, most alcoholics recover from delirium tremens but the mortality rate with inadequate treatment may reach as high as 15%. On the other hand, simple alcohol withdrawal, characterized by insomnia may be managed in a social model setting without medication or on an outpatient detoxification program with sedative-hypnotic medication.

Table 3 summarizes two issues in alcoholism withdrawal. After the acute life-threatening problems and alcohol withdrawal sequelae have been dealt with, emphasis should be placed on getting the individual into aftercare and recovery. The vast majority of alcoholics, in the attempt to return to controlled use of alcohol, will relapse into the active stage of the disease. The focus end point for the treatment of alcoholism should be on abstinence and recovery which focuses on those issues that trigger relapse, and dealing with the negative sequelae of the active stage of their disease. Some of these may be chronic medical problems such as peripheral neuropathy thrombosis or organic brain syndrome. Both require appropriate medical attention.

Psychologically, the alcoholic may experience depression and guilt. Socially, he may manifest serious impairment in family relationships and in personal interaction. In this latter context, the significant social-sexual dysfunction may be evaluated and appropriate therapy initiated. Table 4 demonstrates treatment issues and sequelae that surface early in recovery. In this context, the individual may manifest impairment in a variety of areas including sexual functioning which may be a direct consequence of the psychobiological hormonal impairment secondary to alcoholism. Specific sex therapy or relationship counseling may not be appropriate early in treatment. However, as recovery progresses, factors which contribute to relapse must be dealt with using more individual and family education, as outlined in Table 5.

At this point, one begins assessing the biological basis and reversibility of alcohol induced sexual functioning to get a better idea of what psychopathology is alcohol related and what may occur independent of the alcoholism. For example, we recommend that specific sex therapy for sexual dysfunction not occur until the individual is approximately six months into recovery. Nor do we believe that specific psychotropic medication be initiated for the management of psychiatric disorder such as depression, until the individual is well into recovery, as alcohol-induced depression may disappear completely or an underlying endogenous depression can resurface while the individual is alcohol free and in recovery.

Dr. Apter-Marsh has defined the sexual cycle in both the using and recovering alcoholic. There may be a significant drop in sexual activity during the first 3 to 6 months of recovery.

> Sexuality is likely to be the rawest area of a women's shredded self-esteem. . . . Many alcoholic women have been the victims of sexual abuse and exploitation . . . not just those who have endured loutish husbands . . . we're talking about rape, incest, brutality. While there are no national statistics on the subject, many chemical dependency counselors estimate that nearly 50% of their female clients have been sexually abused as children and teenagers. (Apter-Marsh, 1982)

Our experience indicates that many socio-sexual issues are not identified or discussed individually or with family during the recovery period. Some recovering alcoholics may be tempted to use alcohol to achieve disinhibition in the early recovery period because of sexual concerns, resulting in loss of control and relapse to active alcoholism. Alcohol, although perceived culturally as a sex-enhancing drug via its disinhibiting properties, "is a general central nervous system depressant that has both long and short term effects on sexual functioning. The failure of erection and increased libido described by Shakespeare in Macbeth, for example, is short-term and well known to most men who have attempted to function sexually after excessive alcohol ingestion. People have different thresholds for sexual dysfunction that are related to their blood alcohol level.

Central nervous system effects tend to be more pronounced when levels are rising than when falling. Erectile dysfunctions have more than one cause. Ethanol (ethyl alcohol) impairs spinal reflexes, which causes both decreased sensation and decreased innervation for erection, but it has also been shown to decrease serum testosterone levels" (Buffum, 1981).

One study in which serum testosterone and luteinizing hormones (LH) levels were measured in males before, during and after acute alcohol ingestion showed that, as blood alcohol levels increased, plasma testosterone levels decreased and LH levels increased. The speculation was that the increase in LH levels may have been associated with the increased libido that accompanies acute alcohol ingestion. Decreased serum testosterone, on the other hand, may lead to decreased erection. These effects are usually transient and diminish after the blood alcohol level falls. A similar study was done in women with different results. In this study there was no reduction of serum testosterone or increase in serum LH. There were no consistent effects on progesterone, estradiol, FSH or prolactin.

There are, however, permanent effects related to decreased testosterone levels. A study of normal males given alcohol over a four week period showed that decreased testosterone was coupled with an increase in metabolic clearance. Long-term alcoholics have also been noted to have hyperestrogenemia secondary to alcohol-induced liver damage in which the liver a higher proportion of androgens to estrogens. A combination of decreased testosterone and hyperestrogenemia is probably a cause of the feminization, gynecomastia, sterility, impotence and decreased libido seen in some alcoholic males (Buffum, 1981).

In one study of 17,000 alcoholic males, 8% complained of impotence. In half these cases the impotence was irreversible; in the other half, sexual function returned following several months of abstinence from alcohol. Decreased libido was not mentioned in this study (Buffum, 1981).

Results of a study of 16 non-alcoholic women, who were shown erotic films and given alcohol while being measured with a vaginal photoplethysmograph, indicated that alcohol caused decreased objective signs and increased subjective perception of sexual arousal. This would indicate that vaginal vasocongestion decreases with increasing intoxication, just as does penile erection, its counterpart.

In one study of 44 female chronic alcoholics, 20% said they never experienced orgasm and 36% said they had orgasms less than

5% of the time. It is not clear whether this anorgasmia was related to the adverse physiological effects of alcohol, to the social consequences of alcoholism or to some aspect of the alcoholism-prone personality (Buffum, 1981).

Alcohol combined with other psychoactive drugs such as cocaine is also perceived to have sex enhancing properties. In fact, systematic studies of alcohol and cocaine abusers have demonstrated severe drug-induced sexual dysfunction in many abusers. Cocaine-induced sexual dysfunction may be a factor in seeking treatment for drug abuse. High doses of cocaine, like amphetamine, can also produce sexual behavior that the individual defines as aberrant and unhealthy, ranging from compulsive masturbation, multipartner marathons or sexual abuse of children. This pattern of cocaine-induced aberrant sexual behavior is often produced when the individual combines cocaine with large doses of alcohol which may produce both disinhibition and blackouts (Smith, 1983; Smith, unpublished).

A subgroup of alcoholics also abuse opiates such as heroin, administering it intravenously, or are treated for heroin addiction by oral administration of methadone. The interaction of alcohol and the opiate can impair sexual functioning.

> Heroin is more often related to sexual dysfunction than is methadone, whether in short-term or in long-term. While using methadone, 47% of the males and 67% of the females reported sexual problems, compared to 85% of the males and 87% of the females with sexual difficulty while using heroin. Comparable improvement was noted with specific problems of impotence, libidinal loss and sexual enjoyment while the client was on methadone. (Goldsmith, 1984)

The most effective and powerful group process for recovery from alcoholism is Alcoholics Anonymous. Many recovery groups using the same steps, such as Narcotics Anonymous and Cocaine Anonymous have evolved to deal with other drugs of abuse. The steps are outlined as follows:

1. We admitted that we were powerless over our addiction, that our lives had become unmanageable.
2. We came to believe that a power greater than ourselves could restore us to sanity.

3. We made a decision to turn our will and lives over to the care of God as we understood him.
4. We made a fearless and searching moral inventory of ourselves.
5. We admitted to God, to ourselves and to another human being the exact nature of our wrongs.
6. We were entirely ready to have God remove all these defects of character.
7. We humbly asked Him to remove our shortcomings.
8. We made a list of all persons we had harmed, and became willing to make amends to them all.
9. We made direct amends to such people wherever possible, except when to do so would injure them and others.
10. We continued to take personal inventory, and when we were wrong promptly admitted it.
11. We sought through prayer and meditation to improve our conscious contact as we understood Him, praying only for knowledge of His will for us, and the power to carry it out.
12. Having had a spiritual awakening as a result of those steps, we tried to carry this message to addicts and to practice these principles in all our affairs. (Narcotics Anonymous, 1983)

Often, other types of therapy such as individual counseling, family therapy and sex therapy for persistent sexual dysfunction need to be implemented. Antabuse can be an adjunct to recovery by blocking appreciation of drinking. In the late 1940's disulfiram (Antabuse) was introduced as a therapeutic agent in the treatment of alcoholics. Its mechanism of action is illustrated in Figure 2 (Kanas, 1984).

Early in recovery some alcoholics on Antabuse will describe sexual dysfunction and consider discontinuing Antabuse therapy. For the most part, it is the absence of alcohol with its disinhibiting effects rather than the pharmacological effects of Antabuse which produces the sexual dysfunction. As the disease of alcoholism progresses, so does the socio-sexual impairment.

Studies by Mandell and Miller indicate that individuals who come to alcoholism clinics may not be representative of the general population with regard to social class and general health. The observed rates of occasional sexual dysfunction may be representatives of individuals of similar social background. Also, men who come to alcoholism clinics may have other concurrent undiagnosed

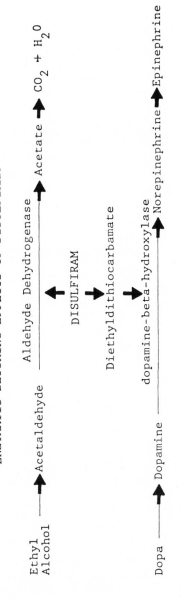

FIGURE 2

ENZYMATIC BLOCKING EFFECTS OF DISULFIRAM

Ethyl Alcohol ⟶ Acetaldehyde ⟶ Aldehyde Dehydrogenase ⟶ Acetate ⟶ $CO_2 + H_2O$

DISULFIRAM

Diethyldithiocarbamate

Dopa ⟶ Dopamine ⟶ dopamine-beta-hydroxylase ⟶ Norepinephrine ⟶ Epinephrine

health problems that increase the risk of dysfunction. Another possibility to be considered is that these subjects may have been consuming more alcohol in the pre-recovery heavy drinking period than they remember. The high rates of dysfunction reported for the period of heaviest drinking may reflect the early onset of alcohol effects on sex function (Mandell, 1983).

Table 6 summarizes the effects of alcohol on sexual function for both male and female by dose (Bush, 1980).

Table 6

EFFECTS OF ALCOHOL ON SEXUAL FUNCTION BY SEX AND AMOUNT OF ALCOHOL*

Small Dose	Moderate Dose	Large Dose	Chronic Alcoholism
WOMEN:			
Release of inhibitions	Fewer or no orgasms	No orgasm	Loss of libido
Feelings of warmth	Decreased quality of orgasm	Lassitude	Loss of menstruation
Increased aggression	Longer foreplay	No lubrication	Frigidity
Increased desire	Decreased lubrication		Infertility
Increased enjoyment of foreplay			
Increased quality of orgasm			
MEN:			
Release of inhibitions	Longer foreplay	Impotence, both erectile and ejaculatory	Loss of libido
Increased aggression	Increased time to erection	Thoughtlessness	Loss of sexual satisfaction
Increased desire	Difficulty in maintaining erection	Unpleasant ejaculation	Erectile impotence
Increased arousal	Uncertain orgasm	Aggressiveness	Decreased testosterone
Control of premature ejaculation	Decreased penile tumescence		Infertility
Decreased penile tumescence			Breast development
			Decreased body hair
			Shriveled testicles

*The amount of alcohol ingestion depends on how strong the drinks are made, how fast they are drunk, the amount of food and drink in the stomach, other drugs taken, weight and age.

Since alcohol abuse and drug and alcohol abuse in combination continue to be substantial problems in our society, it is increasingly important for medical practitioners, psychologists, sex therapists and drug treatment personnel to be aware of the nature and treatment of both addictive disease and related sexual concerns.

REFERENCES

American Psychiatric Association, *Diagnostic and Statistical Manual of Mental Disorders(DSM III)*. 3rd Edition, Washington, D.C.:APA, 1980.

Smith, D.E., "Substance abuse disorders: drugs and alcohol", Lange Publications *Textbook on Psychiatry*, Lange Medical Publications, Los Altos, CA, (1984 publication in progress).

Adler and Kindle, (1981)

Kanas, Nick, "Substance abuse: alcohol," Lange Publications *Textbook on Psychiatry*, Lange Medical Publications, Los Altos, CA, (1984 publication in progress).

Apter-Marsh, The Sexual Behavior of Alcoholic Women While Drinking and During Sobriety. Doctoral Thesis, Institute for the Advanced Study of Human Sexuality, San Francisco, September, 1982.

Sex After Sobriety, (brochure), D.I.N. Publications, Phoenix, 1983.

Buffum, John, et al., "Drugs and sexual function," *Sexual Problems in Medical Practice*, Leif, H., (Ed.), American Medical Association, Chicago, 1981.

Smith, David E., "Treatment considerations with cocaine abusers," *Cocaine: A Second Look*, American Council on Marijuana, Rockville, MD, 1983.

Smith, David E., "Diagnostic treatment and aftercare approaches to cocaine abuse," *Journal of Psychoactive Drugs*, (publication in progress).

Goldsmith, et al., "Methadone folklore: Beliefs about side effects and their impact on treatment," *Human Organization*, (1984, publication in progress).

Narcotics Anonymous, "An Approach to the Fourth Step Inventory," (pamphlet), N.A. World Service Office, Inc., Sun Valley, CA, 1983.

Mandell and Miller, "Male sexual dysfunction as related to alcohol consumption: A pilot study," *Alcoholism: Clinical and Experimental Research*, Vol. 7, No. 1, Winter, 1983.

Bush, Patricia, *Drugs, Alcohol and Sex*. Richard Marek Publishers, NY, 1980.

Returning to Drinking
as a Result of Erectile Dysfunction

Barry W. McCarthy, Ph.D.

Sexual dysfunction, especially erectile problems (impotence), is one of the frequently noted side effects of alcoholism. However, many alcoholic men maintain erectile functioning while drinking. This paper will focus on a syndrome observed in clinical practice, but which has received little research attention in either alcoholism or sex therapy literature. The pattern involves men who have maintained sexual functioning while drinking, attend Alcoholics Anonymous, stop drinking, and begin experiencing erection difficulties. Usually erectile dysfunction has an abrupt onset, but in some cases there is a gradual worsening of erection problems. The typical pattern is loss of erections during intercourse, then loss of erection at point of intromission, difficulty in maintaining erections during the pleasuring/foreplay period, inability to get erections and finally sexual avoidance.

A male can come to believe he has a choice of being a "potent drunk" or an "impotent abstainer," and often chooses the former. The man has few sources of information and counsel since sexuality is not readily discussed in Alcoholics Anonymous nor by physicians or alcoholism counselors. Males put too much of their self-esteem in their penises. The idea of "impotence" connotes more than a difficulty with getting and maintaining erections; it is perceived as a sense of loss of power, masculinity and control. The male goes back to drinking in an effort to regain potency. This is not only self-defeating from the viewpoint of alcoholism, but often does not solve the sexual problem.

When confronted with this situation in clinical practice, the first treatment priority is to control the drinking behavior. The second step is to give information and education about erectile functioning. Males think of erection as automatic, that to be a real man one should be able to get an erection with any woman, any time, and in any situation. Males typically move toward intercourse and orgasm on the first erection. The male client should be made aware that erections are a complex psychophysiological response requiring adequate hormonal, neurological, and vascular functioning; a receptive and responsive psychological state; and a comfortable, cooperative relationship with a partner. A number of physical, psychological, relational, and environmental factors can interfere with erectile functioning. These include alcohol which is a central nervous system depressant. Any negative emotional state (anxiety, depression, anger, or guilt) can interfere with erections. Perhaps the major interference is the man's internal pressure to "perform for his partner", thus taking a "spectator" role. After an initial failure, the male views sex as a performance task rather than being an active, involved partner who sees the sexual experience as a cooperative one where he is free to make requests for additional stimulation. There are a number of professional resources which discuss the psychosocial treatment of erectile dysfunction (Kolodny, Masters & Johnson, 1979; LoPiccolo & LoPiccolo, 1978; McCarthy, 1980; Zilbergeld, 1978).

Most alcoholic men have learned to function sexually in a drinking state. They use alcohol to lower anxieties and inhibitions, to get themselves and their partners into a sexy mood, and to bolster self-confidence. In essence, their sexual learning was state-dependent upon drinking. They are now faced with learning to be comfortable and confident in a new, sober state. This transition can cause temporary erectile difficulty in some men. If they overreact to this temporary problem, they become more self-conscious, become a spectator about their erections and settle into a chronic negative anticipation-performance anxiety erectile dysfunction cycle. What the male needs is information and reassurance that the transition is temporary, and that he must maintain.his sobriety. If the problem worsens or maintains for over three months, referral to a sex therapist would be appropriate.

REFERENCES

Kolodny, R., Masters, W., & Johnson, V. *Textbook of Sexual Medicine*. Boston: Little, Brown, 1979.

LoPiccolo, J. & LoPiccolo, L. (Eds.) *Handbook of Sex Therapy*. New York: Plenum, 1978.

McCarthy, B. Treatment of Secondary Erectile Dysfunction in Males Without Partners. *Journal of Sex Education and Therapy*, 1981, pp. 7, 20-23

Zilbergeld, B. *Male Sexuality*. Boston: Little, Brown, 1978.

The Sexual Behavior
of Alcoholic Women While Drinking
and During Sobriety

Mildred Apter-Marsh, Ph.D.

Both alcohol and sex are concerned with the satisfaction of fundamental urges and have been subjected to infinitely varied codes of behavior, regulations, suppressions and repressions in different communities and phases of civilization (Carver, 1948). Much of the scientific literature on alcoholism tends either to ignore women entirely or to assume that the effects of alcohol on women are the same as they are on men. Similar instances have been evidenced in the literature on human sexuality.

This paper examines and compares the sexual behavior of alcoholic women as it occurred while they were drinking and in sobriety. The sexual behavior patterns of the sample were examined to see what, in fact, they were, and what changes, if any, occurred in them across different time periods. Other sexual characteristics of the sample, such as dreams to orgasm, orgasmic ability, age at first coitus, premarital coitus, extramarital coitus, prostitution, homosexuality, rape and incest, as well as the relationship of alcohol use to sexual experience were examined, and the general sexual behavior of alcoholic women was compared to that of women where alcohol use was not a factor. Two separate sections addressing the first three months of sobriety and treatment recommendations are included also.

PROCEDURES

The sample consisted of 61 white, heterosexual, middle-class, reasonably well-educated recovering alcoholic women, with a mean age of 40 years and a mean length of sobriety of 4.2 years, who were recruited through a "networking" process. Each respondent was required to have a minimum of one year's continuous sobriety, to participate in a private and confidential face-to-face interview, and to answer to their best ability all of the questions asked.

The interview protocol was divided into a drinking and a sexual behavior history, and a sexual dysfunction profile. The drinking history segregated time into three major periods—prior to drinking addictively, while drinking addictively, and during sobriety (which was divided into four sub-phases . . . the first three months, the next nine months, after the first year, and current). The sexual behavior history, based on the Kinsey interview format (Pomeroy, 1982), elicited data on the six chief sources of sexual activity which culminate in orgasm . . . masturbation, nocturnal dreams to climax, heterosexual petting, heterosexual intercourse, homosexual relations and intercourse with animals of other species (Kinsey, 1953). Specific information for each activity was collected for each time period. The sexual dysfunction profile examined what dysfunctions, if any, existed in each time period.

The major focus of this study was twofold: (1) sexual behavior with partners (heterosexual intercourse, homosexual relations and prostitution) and (2) masturbation. Information on nocturnal dreams was considered separately, and the findings on petting to orgasm and zoophilia were of minimal importance. The results of the latter two are not reported in this paper.

Three types of sexual activity were analyzed—sex with partners, masturbation, and a combination of the two. Each activity was viewed from two levels (1) as behavior frequencies and (2) as orgasm frequencies. Each frequency was then examined across two different time perspectives—pre-addiction, addiction and first year of sobriety; and pre-addiction, addiction and total sobriety (which comprised the four sub-phases of sobriety into one period).

SEXUAL BEHAVIOR AND ORGASM OVER TIME

Behavior Frequencies

It is clear that socio-sexual behavior fluctuated greatly during various time periods, while masturbation consistently increased regardless of alcohol use.

Partnered sex. Sex with partners was highest during the addiction period (2.2x week) and lower in total sobriety (1.3x week), but

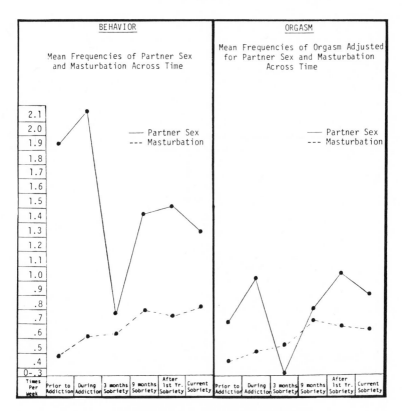

FIGURE 1.   A COMPARISON OF SEXUAL BEHAVIOR AND ORGASM
FREQUENCIES ACROSS SIX INDIVIDUAL TIME PERIODS.

the frequency of activity in total sobriety was not as low as in the first year of sobriety (1.1x week). Women had more sexual activity with partners during addiction than in any other period. Partnered sexual behavior showed significant fluctuation across time, with the lowest frequency occurring in the first three months of sobriety. However, after this period sexual interaction with partners began to climb steadily, so that by total sobriety the women were having almost as much socio-sexual activity as they had had prior to addiction.

Masturbation. When comparing masturbation behavior for pre-addiction, addiction and first year of sobriety and also for pre-addiction, addiction and total sobriety, a different picture emerges. In both analyses, the behaviors across time were not significantly dif-

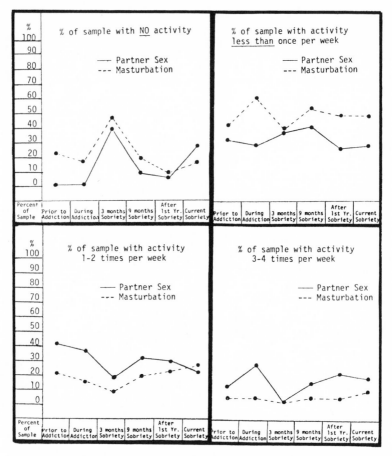

FIGURE 2.   SEXUAL BEHAVIOR FREQUENCIES AS THEY VARY ACROSS
              SIX INDIVIDUAL TIME PERIODS.

ferent. Frequencies gradually and slightly increased over time, but changes were small and the behavior did not appear to be affected by the use or non-use of alcohol. Average frequencies varied only from .5 to .7 times per week.

Partner sex and masturbation combined. Partner sex and masturbation combined were viewed across the same periods as each separate behavior. As in the two time analyses for partnered sex solely, there were significant differences, with the combined activity highest during addiction and lowest in both the first year of sobriety and total sobriety. However, sexual activity was again higher when total sobriety rather than only the first year of sobriety was considered.

Orgasm Frequencies

Across time women became increasingly more orgasmic with socio-sexual activity. Although orgasm was always experienced more through masturbation than through sex with partners, during the drinking periods the gap was even more pronounced. In sobriety, however, the disparity between partnered sexual activity and the ability to orgasm through this source became less, and the percentage of total outlet via partnered sex and the percentage of orgasms from this source were relatively similar—65% and 56% respectively.

Orgasm with partnered sex. Frequency of orgasm in sex with partners was compared across the same time periods as the behavior. When comparing orgasm in the drinking periods vs. the first year of sobriety, the findings were significant. The highest frequency of orgasm with partnered sex occurred during addiction (1.0x week) and the lowest during the first year of sobriety (.5x week). However, when frequency of orgasm in partnered sex was further compared for the drinking periods vs. total sobriety, there were no significant differences. Although orgasm frequencies were still higher during addiction and lower in total sobriety, they were not significantly lower (1.0x week vs. .75x week). In fact, they were almost identical to orgasm frequencies experienced in the pre-addiction period (.71x week).

Partnered sexual behavior is very different when it is adjusted for frequency of orgasm. While women were having more sex with partners during addiction, their ability to orgasm with this behavior in this period was much less—*in essence, they were more active, but less orgasmic in this time period.* The per count number of orgasms in partner sex was greatest during addiction, implying that this was a highly orgasmic phase. However, the frequency of orgasms was actually lower. When the ratio of the level of orgasm to the level of behavior is considered, the subjects were, in fact, more orgasmic in sobriety. *Prior to addiction, the subjects orgasmed with partners 36% of the time. They had twice as much sex with partners during addiction as they had in the first year of sobriety, yet their orgasmic ability was about the same for both periods—47–48%. In total sobriety, however, the subjects were orgasmic 60% of the time that they engaged in sex with partners.*

Orgasm with masturbation. When viewing orgasm with masturbation across the same time sequences, again the frequencies were not significantly different in either analysis. As with the behavior itself, there was a gradual increase over time in both analyses, but changes were small and *frequency of orgasm with masturbation,* contrary to that with socio-sexual activity, *remained relatively constant and did not seem to be affected by using or not using alcohol.* The women were orgasmic with masturbation from 84% of the time in the addiction period to 89–90% during all the other time phases.

Orgasm with partner sex and masturbation combined. Interestingly, when comparing orgasm with the combined activity over the same time perspectives as in the other analyses, there were no significant differences across either time analysis. While there was more combined behavior during addiction and less in sobriety, these differences are only significant when frequency of orgasm is not considered. When orgasm is considered, the differences diminish. Frequency of orgasm with the combined behavior is higher during addiction, but not noticeably higher than it is in sobriety. As in orgasm with sex with partners only, there is a tendency to increase orgasmic ability in the combined activity over time. *Prior to addiction, the subjects were orgasmic 47% of the time; during addiction, 55% of the time; but by total sobriety, they were orgasmic 70% of the time.*

SEXUAL DYSFUNCTION PROFILE

Overall there were no major areas of sexual dysfunction found in this study. Specific questions were asked regarding primary and secondary anorgasmia, dyspareunia, painful noncoital sex, desire phase disorder, and vaginismus across the six time phases. However, questions for this profile required only a "yes" or "no" answer and were less detailed than those used in the sex history. Therefore, although the results in the profile may not coincide with the mean frequencies of sexual behavior and orgasm, in general the findings in the profile do support the findings in the sex history.

More respondents were orgasmically functional in coitus during addiction than prior to addiction (59% vs. 52%). There was a noticeable decrease to 33% in the first three months of sobriety. After the first three months, more women began to be orgasmic during coitus, an ability which increased over time.

The subjects were able to orgasm more frequently and consistently with "other sexual situations" (primarily masturbation) than they were with coitus (85% in prior to addiction, dropping to 75% in the first three months of sobriety, and eventually rising to 97–98% in the later stages of sobriety). The highest level of dyspareunia (painful intercourse) occurred prior to addiction (20%), but this decreased to 3% in the period of sobriety when the data was collected. The incidence of pain in non-sexual situations was less than 2%. There was a very low incidence of vaginismus (involuntary spasmodic contractions of the pubococcygeus muscle); its highest point (less than 7%) was in the during addiction period. Interest and desire in sex remained above 90% in all periods except for the first three months of sobriety, when it dropped to 69%. In the period of sobriety when the data was collected, 100% of the sample indicated they had a desire or interest in sex.

When the women were asked whether they had ever had any sexual concerns across any of the six time periods, 80% responded affirmatively for the drinking phases, 59–64% said "yes" for three of the four sub-phases of sobriety, and 77% said "yes" for current sobriety. The major concerns stated for the drinking periods were promiscuity, guilt, shame, deception, fear of pregnancy, sexual inhibition, and/or sexual repression. For the sobriety periods, however, the concerns most often cited were relationship/intimacy issues—fear of commitment, lack of a partner, disharmony with a partner, communication disintegration—as well as sexual inhibition, desire for more frequency and variety, and lack of assertiveness. Only 3% of the women had a diminished interest or desire in sex.

Sexual dysfunction should not be confused with sexual dissatisfaction. It may be that disinterest in sex and difficulties with sexual arousal and orgasm for alcoholic women result from problems dealing with intimacy in general and relationship disharmony in particular, rather than from sexual dysfunctions such as desire phase disorder or anorgasmia (non-orgasmic).

RELATIONSHIP OF ALCOHOL USE
TO SEXUAL EXPERIENCE

During the drinking periods, the majority of the women always or sometimes used alcohol when they engaged in sex, and a large number of their sexual partners were either heavy drinkers or active alcoholics.

Seventy-nine to eighty per cent (79–80%) of the women reported that when they were drinking, they perceived that alcohol improved their sexual functioning, but not the quality of their orgasms. As length of sobriety increased, however, considerably fewer women maintained this concept, and in the current sobriety time phase, only 2–5% still believed alcohol had improved their ability to function and the quality of their orgasm. While sexual functioning was maximized by the use of alcohol, orgasmic ability was noticeably impaired, and orgasm, when attained, was less intense.

There seems to be little question that for alcoholic women, alcohol acts as a sexual facilitator and enhances sexual arousal and performance, even though sexual physiology indicates otherwise. By following alcoholic women through sobriety over time and comparing both early and later sobriety to the drinking periods, it is found that sexual functioning stabilizes, and orgasmic ability reaches its zenith in the later stages of sobriety.

DREAMS TO ORGASM

Kinsey (1953) said that masturbation and nocturnal sex dreams to the point of orgasm were the activities which provide the best measure of a female's intrinsic sexuality since they require no partners, and hence there is no need to compromise with others. Kinsey's female sample had no more difficulty recalling their dreams to orgasm than did the males, and few women doubted that they reached this stage. The women in the present study indicated that same absence of doubt. Because the data collection format and method used in this study was the same one that Kinsey designed and used (Pomeroy, 1982), the findings for the present study have been appropriately compared to Kinsey's, taking the sizes of the two samples into consideration.

Across time, the number of alcoholic women in this sample who dreamed to orgasm increased, and 52% had their orgasmic dreams in the total sobriety phase.

Overall, 62% of the women in this study dreamed to the point of orgasm at some time in their life; this compares to 20% in Kinsey's sample. An accumulative incidence of 61% of the subjects dreamed to orgasm by age 45; Kinsey found 37%. The peak of activity for the respondents occurred between 30–39 years of age; in Kinsey's group, it was 40–50 years of age. Thirty-nine per cent (39%) of the women in this study experienced orgasmic dreams not more than 1–6 times in their life; Kinsey found 25%. In this sample, 29% regularly experienced over 5 dreams to orgasm per year; Kinsey had 8%. In each instance of comparison, the women in this study show a greater tendency to experience orgasmic dreams than did Kinsey's group.

OTHER SEXUAL CHARACTERISTICS OF THE SAMPLE

Space does not permit further detail of the other interesting sexual characteristics found in this study, particularly the variety and degree of sexual encounters experienced by these women and the role which alcohol played in their sexual lives.

In summary, however, *the alcoholic women in this study appear to be "intrinsically sexual."*

Almost two-thirds of the women dreamed to the point of orgasm at least once in their life. One hundred per cent (100%) masturbated at least once, and almost half by the age of twelve. Ninety-eight per cent (98%) reached orgasm at some point during their life. Twenty per cent (20%) experienced coitus by the age of fifteen. Eighty-two per cent (82%) had intercourse prior to marriage. The median number of sexual partners was 26. About two-thirds participated to some degree in extramarital intercourse. Fifteen per cent (15%) engaged in prostitution to a limited degree. Twenty-eight per cent (28%) had an occasional homosexual experience after the age of fifteen. Nearly 50% of the women had been raped or forced into having sex. Slightly more than 25% reported sexual activity with a family member. Though some of these women had broad sexual experience, interestingly their behavior is not radically different from that of other women in recent sexuality studies whose use of alcohol was not examined (Hunt, 1974; Wolfe, 1980).

Varied sexual experiences such as those reported can provoke feelings of not conforming to society's prescribed female behaviors which are still, for many, prerequisites for social approval and love.

Being a sexually active woman, even in today's society, is not sanctioned as "traditional womanly behavior." It may appear on the surface that these women engaged in sexual behavior with careless abandon. In the majority of cases, however, the reverse was true. Their sexual activities left them feeling unwomanly, unwanted and unworthy. Schuckit (1972) states that "promiscuous" would describe only a small proportion of alcoholic women if promiscuity was defined as "indiscriminate" sexual indulgence, and the present study supports Schuckit. This author believes the subjects were not "indiscriminate," but rather sexually motivated as evidenced by intrinsic sexual factors: dreams to orgasm, masturbation frequencies, and orgasmic ability, etc.

FIRST THREE MONTHS OF SOBRIETY

The first three months of sobriety is a time of great importance in the addiction recovery process, a time when readjustments in all phases converge: physical, psychological, spiritual, social and sexual. *By examining the first three months separately from the following nine months of sobriety, it became obvious in this study that women's sexuality in their earliest phase of sobriety underwent considerable change.* For example, when compared to the addiction period, this early phase of sobriety showed a major decline in both socio-sexual activity and in orgasm from this source, as well as many changes in masturbation. Of the six time periods, only this one showed a marked increase in the number of women who had neither socio-sexual nor masturbation activity. During this period, one-third of the women who had been masturbating stopped completely when they ceased drinking. But by the end of six months of sobriety, 85% of this group had resumed the activity. On the other hand, one-half of the women, when they stopped drinking, increased their masturbation frequency from what it had been.

In this study, many women spoke of their anxieties about their sexuality in this early period of sobriety. Some had felt their bodies had "shut down" and were fearful that they would be sexually impaired permanently. Others had been distraught over past sexual behavior when drinking and felt deep guilt, shame and anger. Some were concerned because they were having sexual dreams and fantasies which they felt were wrong, and a further indication of their unworthiness. And others felt sexual stirrings in an uninebriated state for the first time and were frightened by such unfamiliar physical sensations.

Other studies on alcoholic women have, however, reported incidences of desire dysfunction and primary and secondary anorgasmia (Hammond, 1980; Murphy, 1980; *Sexual Medicine Today*). For the women in this study, sexual desire was consistent, except for a slight decline in the first three months of sobriety, and the majority remained orgasmic throughout all periods.

The conflicting nature of reports from other studies may stem from the time period in which the information was gathered. If data is collected in the early periods of recovery, there may, indeed, be indications of loss of libido, sexual inhibition, and a decline in orgasmic ability. In later stages of sobriety, however, these problems usually diminish. *It is, therefore, important not to interpret data collected in periods of early sobriety as indicators of extensive sexual dysfunction. If given sufficient time, symptoms of such dysfunction will usually spontaneously disappear for a majority of the cases.*

TREATMENT RECOMMENDATIONS

Alcohol affects the sexuality of alcoholic women in different ways at different times. It can lower sexual inhibitions and facilitate socio-sexual interaction, as well as impair orgasmic ability and promote feelings of unwomanliness, inadequacy and low self-esteem. It can act as an anesthetizer on the one hand and as an enhancer on the other. However, the effects of alcohol on the sexuality of female alcoholics do not appear to be permanent or fixed.

In the early stages of sobriety, vast changes do occur in all life situations. Physical toxicity begins to diminish and, in some cases, can take months before it dissipates entirely. Emotional "toxicity" as well needs time to recover: psychological, spiritual and social growth and change happen slowly. It is imperative to recognize that many alcoholic women in the early stages of recovery are unaware of the snail-like pace of rehabilitation and seek to have all of their problems solved immediately once they are sober.

The following recommendations are offered when treatment of the sexual concerns of alcoholic women are being considered.

1. Alcoholic women's sexuality undergoes its greatest alterations in the earliest stages of sobriety, and for many, sexual functioning

with both self and partners temporarily ceases. The advent of such changes can create unnecessary fears and anxieties. It is important, therefore, to recognize the presence of such concerns in this fragile period and to provide these women with sexual information to help alleviate their fears and, at the same time, to endorse their femininity and worthiness as women. They need to know in early sobriety that sexual dysfunction symptoms may appear, but that such "dysfunction" will very likely disappear in time. They need to anticipate, without fear, sexual changes which may occur in these early phases. They need to know that their womanliness is not under attack; that their sexual bodies and psyches are merely in the throes of convalescence, just as are all other components of their lives. They need to be reassured that much of what they may be experiencing will most likely reverse itself in time.

2. Many alcoholic women suffer deep feelings of guilt, shame and anger about their non-sanctioned sexual behavior which elevates their sense of unworthiness and lack of self-esteem. They need to learn how to evaluate their sexual behavior when they were drinking. For example, their husbands were likely to have been heavy drinkers or alcoholics, and extramarital sex may have been a reaction to an unhappy, nonsexual marriage. Further, as women they probably received little schooling on "how to say no" and this, combined with an intrinsic sexual nature, may have precipitated activity which was unwanted or unfulfilling. They need to ventilate their feelings and concerns about their sexual experiences: sexual anger at men or at themselves, disenchantment with or disapproval of their own sexual behavior (whether sanctioned or not) and distorted guilt and fears. It is important that alcoholic women learn positive and reinforcing ways to express their sexuality without the aid of alcohol.

3. Many alcoholic women have been raped or forced into having sex or have experienced sexual activity with a family member. These kinds of sexual experiences can produce negative influences on later sexual adjustment. It is important that they be addressed in recovery so that their feelings about such experiences can be thoroughly processed.

4. Therapists should not confuse sexual dissatisfaction with sexual dysfunction. Many alcoholic women suffer with intimacy problems in general—lack of relationships, lack of a partner, difficulty in establishing new relationships, or disharmony in existing relationships—all of which can effect sexual interacting and, if not resolved, can be threatening to sobriety.

5. Because of the interrelationship of sex and alcohol, women in early sobriety have frequently been advised by alcoholism counselors and AA members to refrain from sex. The likelihood of alcoholics totally relinquishing their sexuality in order to maintain sobriety is not very probable. Censuring sex is not the answer, and, in fact, may be a greater threat than an asset in maintaining sobriety. "Being sexual" is not the problem. The problem is knowing how to express sexuality, either alone or with a partner, without the aid of alcohol and for the appropriate reasons.

6. It is important to consider the length of sobriety of the alcoholic before commencing sexual counseling. Toxicity, both physical and emotional, may still be present. Patients need to be evaluated on an individual basis, but it probably would be best to wait at least six to eight months before beginning specific treatment for sexual dysfunctions such as anorgasmia, desire phase disorders, etc.

7. Many alcoholism rehabilitation programs do not address sexuality issues in early recovery because sex, usually translated to mean sexual intercourse with a partner, is believed to be less important than other life situations which need attention. However, it is important to recognize that the issues mentioned are all sexuality concerns, that such sexual concerns occur during the very early stages of sobriety, and that recovering alcoholic women need early access to information which can help alleviate their fears and anxieties about their sexual selves. Appropriate education in early recovery sets the stage for later sobriety. Sexuality needs to be addressed in early alcoholism treatment. If it is ignored, it leaves many questions unanswered and many painful memories unresolved, promotes unnecessary sexual concerns, and delays the construction of the foundations of alcoholism rehabilitation: self-worth and self-esteem.

CONCLUSION

Sexual behavior of alcoholic women changes with their use and non-use of alcohol. These changes are not fixed or permanent. Information collected in a single phase of addiction or sobriety may very likely indicate extensive sexual dysfunction when, in actuality, if given enough time, there is none. Likewise sexual behavior in the during addiction period is not a true indicator of the sexual behavior of "alcoholics." It is most important to recognize that sexuality changes across the different time phases, and no one phase represents the alcoholic in totality.

It is important to cease applying a tunnel-vision interpretation of "penis/vagina" sex to sexuality and tossing this interpretation lightly aside without further consideration of the much broader scope of sexuality. It is time to acknowledge sexuality and accept it as a major component of being human, healthy and normal. It is becoming more apparent that unresolved sexuality issues can be a major threat to the recovering alcoholic's sobriety (Mandell, 1982; Rosellini, 1982; *Sexual Medicine Today*; and Talbott, 1982.) Women in sobriety need not only to acknowledge but to celebrate their intrinsic sexuality and to learn what their sexual options are without alcohol. Opening this door in early recovery is neither the primary nor the sole solution to recidivism. But recovering alcoholic women who gain further insights into their sexual selves will better understand, accept and respect who they are—women first and alcoholics after—which, in the long run, can only help foster a more secure sobriety and a more rewarding life, both sexual as well as non-sexual.

BIBLIOGRAPHY

Carver, A. The interrelationship of sex and alcohol. *The International Journal of Sexology*, 1948, 2(2), pp. 78–81.

Hammond, D., Jorgensen, G., & Ridgeway, D. *Sexual Adjustment of Female Alcoholics*. Unpublished manuscript, Univ. of Utah, Salt Lake City, 1980.

Hunt, M. *Sexual Behavior in the 1970's*. Chicago: Playboy Press, 1974.

Kinsey, A., Pomeroy, W., & Martin, C. *Sexual Behavior in the Human Male*. Philadelphia: W.B.Saunders Co., 1948.

Kinsey, A., Pomeroy, W., Martin, C. & Gebhard, P. *Sexual Behavior in the Human Female*. Philadelphia: W.B. Saunders Co., 1953.

Mandell, L. & North, S. Sex roles, sexuality and the recovering woman alcoholic: Program issues, *Journal of Psychoactive Drugs*, 1982, 14 (1–2), pp. 163–166.

Murphy, W., Coleman, E., Hoon, E. & Scott, C. Sexual dysfunction and treatment in alcoholic women. *Sexuality and Disability*, 1980, *3(4)*, pp. 240–255.

Pomeroy, W., Flax, C. & Wheeler, C. *Taking a Sex History*. New York, Free Press, 1982.

Rosellini, G. Is there sex after sobriety? The quandary of the recovering woman. *Alcoholism, the National Magazine*, October, 1982, pp. 31–32.

Schuckit, M. Sexual disturbance in the woman alcoholic. *Medical Aspects of Human Sexuality*, September, 1972, pp. 44–65.

Sexual medicine for alcoholics. *Sexual Medicine Today*, June, 1981, 5(6), pp. 26–27.

Talbott, G. Douglas, M.D., Director, Alcohol and Drug Programs, Ridgeview Institute, Smyrna, Georgia. Personal conversation, March 6–10, 1982.

Wolfe, L. The sexual profile of that Cosmopolitan Girl. *Cosmopolitan Magazine*, September, 1980, pp. 254–257; 263–265.

Assessment of Sexual Functioning

Robert W. Fuller, M.A.

INTRODUCTION

The alcoholism and drug abuse field has at last begun to seriously consider its responsibility for dealing with sexual behaviors and problems of its clients. However, a sober scrutiny within the medical/psychiatric community reveals that the average counselor, commonly believed to be an authority on mental health and human sexuality, is no more able to deal with sexual issues than many nonprofessionals. The average counselor in training or in practice tends to be no more knowledgeable or sexually experienced than his age peers and may in fact be less open in matters concerning sexual activity (GAP, 1973).

Since little comprehensive training in human sexuality is provided in undergraduate or graduate level programs in the behavioral sciences, most professional counselors has little or no formal education on basic sexual activity, physiology or functioning. And yet sexual problems are prevalent among clients of alcoholism workers. Further training is needed for counselors in assessing, identifying, evaluating and treating sexual disorders, especially in alcohol or drug abuse patients. This paper is designed to contribute to the counselor's education in matters of sexual behavior, and particularly to help obtain appropriate sexual information from the client in the diversity of treatment situations where it is relevant.

The same principles of clinical interviewing that apply elsewhere in therapy are appropriate in assessing sexual functioning.

Since alcoholism can co-exist with other medical and psychiatric problems, such as depression, psychosis, liver disease, diabetes, etc., all of which might contribute to sexual dysfunctions, a sound differential diagnosis is important. Also at times sexual problems mask underlying psychological conflicts which should be detected and understood before focusing primarily on the sexual problems

49

themselves. This paper seeks to aid the counselor in identifying these issues.

THE RELEVANCE OF DIAGNOSIS

An accurate diagnosis is the single most important factor in any treatment process, and especially in dealing with sexual functioning due to the many diverse psychological and biological stressors that produce identical symptoms. It is estimated that 15-25% of sexual problems are physiologically based in the non-alcoholic population. Undoubtedly, this figure is higher for alcoholics.

For example, a number of medical complications are associated with alcoholism that may result in sexual problems: endocrine conditions, i.e., diabetes, pituitary, adrenal, and thyroid disorders; vascular and cardiac problems; neurological deficiencies; hepatic or kidney diseases; nutritional deficiencies and urologic disorders. The organic factors contributing to sexual problems must be differentiated to determine an appropriate diagnosis.

Other psychiatric problems contributing to sexual disorders should also be assessed, such as, depression (often resulting in inhibited sexual desire, ISD); stress and anxiety, panic or phobic disorders; obsessive/compulsive behavior; and passive-aggressive behavior.

Finally, complications resulting from medications must also be differentiated to arrive at an accurate diagnosis. Medications that may result in sexual disorders are antihypertensives, adrenergic-receptor blockers, antipsychotic or antidepressant drugs, hypnotics and antianxiety agents, amphetamines, narcotics, endocrine medication, and especially Antabuse. It is estimated that 10-50% of males using Antabuse experience some degree of periodic impotence (Kaplan, 1979).

Therefore, it is important in the treatment process to determine the medical, psychiatric and/or medication-related etiologies for sexual problems prior to treatment of the sexual complaints. An accurate diagnosis is critical to this process. The method recommended for the assessment of sexual functioning involves a clinical interview, supplemented when necessary by information derived from a physical examination, laboratory tests and special diagnostic procedures used in sexual counseling. Medical and psychological aspects of the assessment process are incorporated into the diagnosis. The cornerstones for the assessment are traditional psychosexual dysfunctions as outlined in the *Diagnostic and Statistical Manual* of the American Psychiatric Association (DSM-III, APA, 1980), the triphasic concept of sexual response (Kaplan, 1974), and Masters and Johnson's sex therapy approaches (Masters and Johnson, 1970).

This paper is divided into the following sections: the Information derived from the psychosexual assessment, and the Methodology for taking the assessment. The paper seeks to serve as a working guide for clinicians in assessing sexual problems in alcoholic clients.

INFORMATION

In order to deal with sexual problems and to formulate a treatment plan, the alcoholism counselor must identify if there is a problem, what is the chief complaint, establish an accurate diagnosis, and determine etiology. To do so, a differential diagnosis between organic and psychogenic causes, and an analysis of the psychosocial elements of the issue are necessary. The basic questions for an alcoholism counselor to address in the counseling process, regardless of the treatment setting, are:

1. Is there a sexual problem?
2. What is the problem? The diagnosis? Its etiology?
3. Is the problem primary or secondary to other psychological and/or medical problems? Is it alcohol-induced only and perhaps spontaneously reversible? Are there deeper psychological causes of the problem? What are their severity?
4. What are the relational issues involved in the sexual problems?

Each of these questions will be dealt with in the following section. The methodology of questioning for a sexual problem assessment will be addressed in subsequent sections.

Is There a Problem?

Since alcoholism impacts on all aspects of one's life, including physically, psychologically, socially, relationally, and spiritually, it can be assumed that most alcoholics presenting themselves in treatment will have experienced some sexual problems. However, it cannot be assumed that all individuals who say they have a sexual problem necessitate treatment for that problem, nor can it be assumed that those reporting no sexual problems shouldn't be treated for sexual issues. Psychosexual complaints may be a result of minor anxieties, lack of knowledge, inexperience, etc., and thus simple, brief support, information and reassurance may be adequate to resolve the "problem." Sexual problems may be a reflection of the more primary problems of unconscious insecurities, latent anxieties, separation stress, rejection sensitivity, obsessive-compulsive behaviors, depression, neurotic conflicts, etc. Thus, the first question is whether there is truly a problem or if it is a displacement of other emotional or relationship problems. If that is the case, usually reassurance about one's sexual normalcy is sufficient to deal with the sexual complaint. Of course, to determine normalcy of one's behavior, a clear picture of the current sexual functioning is necessary.

CHART I
DECISION-MAKING IN THE ASSESSMENT OF SEXUAL FUNCTIONING*

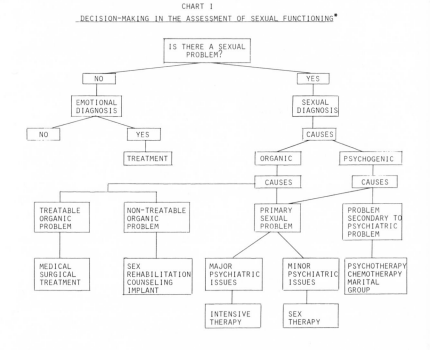

* ADAPTED FROM KAPLAN, THE EVALUATION OF SEXUAL DISORDERS, 1983.

What is the Problem? Its Etiology?

The key questions in determining diagnosis are:

1. What phase of the sexual response cycle is impaired: desire, excitement, or orgasm phase (Kaplan's Tri-Phasic concept of Sexual Functioning, 1979)?
2. What is the degree, extent, nature and severity of the impairment?
3. How does that affect the individual? The couple?

Determining etiology is critical to the differential diagnostic process. What is the cause? Is its etiology organic or psychogenic? With alcoholics, it is speculated that 15-25% of sexual problems have a medical/organic basis, especially those over the age of 40. To help determine cause, the following questions should be asked: Is the problem related to specific circumstances? If it is situational organic etiology can be ruled out, eliminating the need for further medical and laboratory workup.

Does the problem have a high/low probability for organicity, such as impotence in male alcoholics, dyspareunia in both sexes, vaginismus, secondary ejaculatory incompetence, or secondary anorgasmia? The following sexual problems are typically not associated with physical etiology: primary ejaculatory incompetence, primary anorgasmia in females, homosexuality, paraphilias, situational inhibited sexual desire, sexual phobias and avoidance.

Further, a determination should be made if the sexual issues may be reversible. What is the probability that the problem will spontaneously resolve itself over time? Examples of reversible conditions are: loss of sexual desire as a result of endocrine deficiencies, tumors, depression, or stress; inadequate female lubrication due to estrogen deficiencies; impotence resulting from the administration of antihypertensive medication; penile vascular impairment; vaginal obstructions; dyspareunia resulting from infections, endometriosis, hymenal tags, episiotomy scarring, hernia, or herpes; or orgasm phase disorders from vitamin deficiencies, viral infections, MAO inhibitor medications.

The following problems are likely to be irreversible without addressing the primary diagnostic issue: impotence or anorgasmia resulting from diabetes, small vessel arteriosclerosis, vaginal atrophy, degenerative neurological disease, central nervous system and surgical trauma, or renal dialysis.

A general rule is that primary sexual disorders are likely to have a psychogenic etiology provided the person does not suffer from congenital abnormalities, or physical trauma. If the individual has experienced successful sexual functioning for a period of time and later experiences a sexual disorder (secondary disability), the possibility of both organic and/or psychogenic etiology should be explored.

Other critical questions are if there is any illness that could cause the problem? Has the illness/injury been treated? Are medications for the illness causing sexual side-effects? Further, can the sexual problems be cured? How extensive is the sexual problem?

Primary vs. Secondary to a Psychiatric Problem

Clearly, alcoholics and their partners experience a range of emotional disorders: depression, phobias, obsessive-compulsive behavior, stress, anxiety disorders, personality disorders, retardation, etc. Therefore, the following questions should be addressed in the assessment process. Is there a psychiatric disorder? What is it? Is it appropriate to deal with the sexual problems? Can they benefit from psychiatric treatment first? Is the person suicidal/homicidal? Which came first—the sexual symptom or the psychiatric disorder? Is the sexual problem a product of or a defense against the psychiatric problem? Is the psychiatric problem alcohol-induced? Will the symptom spontaneously reverse itself over time?

For example, Dr. Harold Lief (Lief, 1982), estimates that "30-40% of sexually dysfunctional patients improvement will occur without major psychodynamic changes." Of the remaining 60%, 10% should have individual psychotherapy, 20% marital counseling, and 30% a combination of marital and sex therapy.

Once the above determinations have been made (Is there a problem? Is it psychogenic or organic? A psychiatric-related disorder?), the immediate and deeper psychological causes of the problem and their severity and prognosis for resolution should be dealt with.

> These cognitive and emotional processes are specifically instrumental in disrupting the individual's erotic feelings and sexual reflexes and so produce the symptom in the here and now . . . . Psychosexual symptoms may be characterized as

the resultant of the interaction of these immediate psychobe-havioral antecedents and the physiologic phase of the sexual response which they disrupt.

The success of treatment depends on eliminating or modifying the immediate, currently operating psychobehavioral anteced-ents which are impairing the patient's functioning. This is the crucial ingredient for cure and the basic strategy of sex ther-apy. (Kaplan, 1979)

Deeper psychologic causes of the sexual problem may involve re-lationship issues or intrapsychic causes for either the alcoholic or co-alcoholic. In some cases, sexual symptoms are reflective of deeper needs to avoid sexuality. The emotional/neurotic roots, and their psychodynamics should be questioned. Are deeper negative re-ligious or cultural messages causing the problem? Are these factors conscious or unconscious? Examples of deeper psychological roots include: long-standing fears of failure/success, ambivalence to-wards the opposite sex, pathologic relationships with parents, nega-tive sociocultural attitudes about sex, neurotic processes, destruc-tive sexual "scripting," or sexual trauma. Are these deeper causes minor/severe?

What Are the Relational Issues?

Whenever there are two individuals, both are the patient (Masters and Johnson, 1970). Both partners are always involved in the prob-lem and hopefully the treatment. It inevitably involves a faulty rela-tional system and inadequate sexual interactions. This is especially true in a deteriorating alcoholic relationship. However, there are some exceptions: an individual may be impotent with his current partner, and all other prior partners. The dyadic elements may con-tribute to intrapsychic origins of the problems. Therefore, it is im-portant to ask the following questions. What is the relationship sys-tem? Is the problem related to the current partner? Are specific relationship problems contributing to the sexual issues, such as communication impairment, lack of sexual attraction, unresolved power struggles, parental transferences, contractual issues, inti-macy/commitment disorders, partner psychopathology, or irrecon-cilable marital incompatibility.

Finally, the unique needs of the single alcoholic client should be explored, such as socialization needs, defensive rationalizations about the lack of a partner, feelings of loneliness/depression, confused sexual identity, lack of sexual confidence, shyness, frustration, and "the widower's syndrome" resulting from infrequent/nonexistent sexual activity ("If you don't use it, you lose it").

HOW TO TAKE A SEX PROBLEM HISTORY

There is considerable controversy in the substance abuse field about when to treat the recovering person for sexual problems. However, there should be little doubt that from the onset of treatment, some form of sexual problem history should be taken. The details of the problem can be filled in over the treatment process. From day one of treatment, when the psychosocial and medical history is taken, basic questions about the patient's sexual life should also be asked, such as, "It often happens that alcoholics and their partners experience some form of sexual problems, probably as a result of continued alcohol abuse. Which of these problems have you and your partner experienced . . . ? What chief complaint do you have about your sexual relationship? Was there ever a time when you had no sexual problems?" The purpose of these questions is to determine the nature, and chronology (history) of the chief complaints.

Other sexual performance issues to be addressed in the intake process are: "Are you satisfied with the sexual adjustment in your marriage? Do you think your partner is satisfied? Have you discussed these problems with a professional counselor, doctor, etc.? How frequently do you and your spouse have intercourse presently? Formerly? How do you both feel about that frequency? What changes have you seen in your sex life over the past year? 5 years?"

If problems seems to arise from this initial sex problem information, a decision should be made immediately regarding the severity of the problem, its impact on the total recovery of the person, the relationship issues that might interfere with achieving sobriety, the appropriateness of dealing with these sexual issues in the current treatment system, the ability of the patient to address sexual issues, the clinical capability of the treatment team, and the appropriate stage of treating the sexual problems.

Once a determination has been made that this is the appropriate time and setting to deal with the sexual problems, a detailed description of the patient's historic and current sexual experiences/ problems and relationship interactions should be derived. This sexual status examination should include an assessment of medical status.

Medical Status Examination

Laboratory tests and a physical examination to screen medical causes of sexual symptoms should be performed: nocturnal penile tumescence (NPT) monitoring, tests of thyroid deficiency states, serum testosterone, serum prolactin, estrogen, and follicle stimulating hormone level tests, penile blood pressure and penile blood flow examination, the glucose tolerance test, and hepatic disease tests. A physical examination of the genitalia should be conducted by a skilled physician, particularly if the person complains of sexual discomfort and pain, lack of lubrication, vaginismus, or an unconsummated marriage. The gynecologic examination should explore conditions such as multiple sclerosis, alcoholic neuropathy, tabes dorsalis, malnutrition with vitamin deficiencies, irregular lesions in the spinal cord, diabetes mellitus, intact or rigid hymen, clitoral problems, vulvitis, herpes genitales type 2, dermatologic conditions, operative scarring, urethritis, pelvic inflammatory disease, a congenital shortened vagina, endometriosis, ovarian pathology, lower bowel disease, or pelvic congestion.

The urologic examination for the male should concentrate on blood pressure, surgical incisions, examination of the lower urinary tract, abdomen, perineum, external genitalia, inguinal areas for herpes, a digital rectal examination, anal sphincter tone, prostate gland, reflexes, cutaneous sensations, motor strength, and peripheral pulses. Semen analysis should be performed by laboratory examination of an ejaculate, including volume, sperm count, motility, quality of activity, percentage mobile, and morphology.

If impotence is the chief complaint, the following pathology should be explored: local penile anatomic abnormalities, neurogenic factors (i.e., spinal cord injury), vasculogenic factors, endocrine-related problems (testicular size and testosterone levels, prolactin), and diabetes. Finally, the person conducting the assessment should carefully explore the use of medications that may interfere with sexual functioning.

Since gender identity disorders (transsexual), although prevalent in alcoholism, rarely involve organic etiology, and as such would involve primarily a psychosexual history, a medical/laboratory examination is rarely indicated. The same is true for egodystonic homosexuality.

Psychosexual History

Up to this point, the paper has addressed the medical and physical aspects of the sexual problem; the focus will turn to the family and psychosocial/sexual history issues. It is important for a complete picture of the client to be presented, including socialization patterns; racial, ethnic, and religious background that might influence sexual functioning; sex education issues; and sexual functioning, past and present. The history should provide information on all sexual involvements, both successful or unsuccessful, heterosexual/homosexual. Early sexual "failures" should be uncovered.

The relationship should be assessed as well. This part of the process is designed to assess deeper problems in the couple's interactions and to determine if these issues are symptomatic of the sexual problems or vice versa. The evaluation of the relationship occurs by observing their interactions, noting the feelings evoked in the couple and in the clinician. For example, most healthy, loving couples give off a feeling of well-being. A dysfunctional, disharmonious couple conveys a feeling of discomfort, or perhaps annoyance. Although the clinician does not, of course, take sides for or against the couple or either partner, he should be sensitive to the feeling tone conveyed in the interview for these feelings are important diagnostic tools.

The couple's interactions should be assessed. Are the following signs present: cooperation, support, anger, power struggles, ambivalence, anxiety, coldness, affection, etc. These signs are conveyed via eye contact, body movement, and conversation. How does the couple communicate? Are the verbalizations adequate? Is there a level of intimacy, sensitivity, empathy with each other? To what extent might the communication problems influence the sexual issues? How is that sexual complaint presented—"All our problems are her fault. I'm blameless." "I'll do anything to make it better." Is one partner self-demeaning, cold and withdrawn from the problem, or supportive and encouraging? What power struggles are witnessed? What is the evidence for contractual disappointment, acting out, affairs, etc.

The reality status of the relationship should also be assessed, including their dating history, how long they lived together/been married. What are their feelings about each other? Do they love one another? What interest/commitment is there to make the relationship work? Commitment is a very powerful tool for the clinician in the therapy process and should be assessed. "How committed are you? To what extent are you willing to change? Do you picture yourself together as a couple in one year? Five years? On a scale of 1–10 with 10 being almost heaven, how do you rate the emotional health of the relationship? Sexual life? How often do you argue/fight? About what? What goes on when you fight? Violence? If you were a tailor designing a couple, how would you describe the fit of your relationship? Who's in charge? Who makes decisions? How does the other person feel about decision-making?" Throughout these questions the clinician is seeking to find out if there are signs of deeper psychodynamic conflicts.

The specific psychosexual issues in a relationship should be assessed: Is there performance anxiety, pressure to perform, unrealistic expectations of sex, spectatoring, sexual avoidance/aversion? Is there sexual acting out, aggressive sexual demands, critical attitudes displayed, a nonsupportive partner, information and knowledge gaps, technique problems, etc.

All of this information can be compiled by a skilled clinician in a one hour session. More involved cases may require 2–3 sessions, especially if there is a combination of organic and psychogenic etiology of the sexual problems. If an organic basis is suspected, prompt referral for a physical examination and laboratory testing should be made, followed up by a debriefing session with the referring counselor. With alcoholics, since a high probability of a medical overlay exists with most sexual problems, a medical workup should usually be recommended. The cost for routine serum testosterone level workups is minimal when performed with other routine laboratory tests and should probably be added to the battery of tests performed by an inpatient unit.

If psychogenic and/or relationship issues are involved, separate sessions with each partner may be appropriate to explore individual sexual histories, "secrets," affairs, etc. Has one partner decided to leave, is homosexual/bisexual, finds his partner sexually unattractive? These individual sessions may require from 30–90 minutes depending on the degree and complexity of the pathology, and the severity of the communication problems.

After the couple is seen separately a "roundtable" debriefing should be held. The summation includes the clinician's clear assessment of the problem, its complexity, each partner's involvement, interim conclusions, prognosis, and some note of optimism, regardless of the problem severity. Reassurance, support and encouragement are important from the onset. If no physical basis for the problem is apparent, the clinician should so indicate in a reassuring manner. This summation should enhance the clinician/client relationship, establishing a mutual problem-solving attitude. It should be sensitive to their anxiety levels. It should impart information and specific suggestions for change—a road map to further counseling.

If the problem is organic and/or irreversible, such information should be conveyed in a sensitive, supportive manner. Again, some note of optimism about what can be done should be conveyed.

The roundtable should end with specific recommendations for immediate change. If the couple will be continuing on with that counselor, suggestions between appointments should be given. If a referral is made, the clinician should provide recommendations and assistance up to the point the couple is seen by the other agent. Finally, if addressing the sexual issues is postponed until later in the recovery process, interim suggestions should be offered, such as how to overcome anxiety about sex, temporarily limiting sexual involvement, techniques to enhance communication and openness, intimacy building, etc. The bottom line is, however, that these recommendations should enhance and not threaten the growing potential for sobriety and recovery.

The Format of a General Sex History

The format of a general sex history is a combination of the work of GAP (1973), Masters and Johnson (1970), and Hartman (1972) and can be used with both males and females, except where it is listed specifically by sex. The questions are asked in the language of the client determined as the counselor proceeds through the psychosocial intake. Throughout the interview the counselor should adapt the process to the dynamics of the alcoholic relationship, the stage of recovery of the alcoholic, and the history of relapses.

Not all segments of the history are appropriate; the counselor must be selective in history-taking, using the rule, "If you are not going to use the information derived, don't ask about it." This format assumes the basic identifying data has been derived from the psychosocial intake, such as age, history of addiction, parental and family information, sociologic and psychologic data. The following questions are in outline form, providing the key phrase or topic to be addressed. It is left to the skill of the counselor to phrase the question in a non-threatening, therapeutic manner.

I. Childhood sexuality
   A. Family attitudes about sex, nudity, modesty; parental discussions about sex; siblings, close relatives; peers.
   B. Other influences about sex: ethnic, religious, cultural.
   C. Learning about sex: parents (questions asked/answered; at what age; feelings about it); information volunteered by family; explanations by each parent about sex play, pregnancy, birth, intercourse, masturbation, nocturnal emissions, menstruation, homosexuality.
   D. Sexual experimentation: first sight of nude body of same sex/opposite sex; feelings about it; genital self-stimulation; other solitary sexual activities; first sexual play/exploration; sexual activity with older persons; seeing animals in coitus/giving birth.
   E. Parental sex: intercourse
   F. Childhood sexual theories and myths about conception/birth, genitals, etc.

II. Onset of adolescence
   A. In girls: preparation for menstruation (informant, nature of information, age given, feelings); first period (duration, frequency, reaction, hygenic method); other body changes; erotic responsiveness.
   B. In boys: preparation for adolescence; ages of changes; erotic responsiveness.

III. Contraceptive background
   A. Earlier experiences
   B. Present utilization and effects on sexual response

IV. Heterosexual experiences
   A. Pre-adolescent/adolescent/dating experiences (age, sex, frequency, number, techniques).
   B. Involvement with kin (parent, siblings); reactions; problems.
   C. Dating (number before first sexual encounter, sexual preplay, nudity, attitudes about premarital coitus).
   D. Premarital (number, age, sex, ethnic or racial background, marital status, prostitutes, frequency, tech-

      niques, effects on later marriage, contraception, orgasm, erections).

   E. Engagements (same as D)

   F. Other premarital experiences (rape, pregnancy, births, abortions, coital positions, preferences for light/ darkness/nudity, general sexual preference).

   G. Orgastic experiences (nocturnal emissions or orgasm during sleep, via masturbation, necking and petting, intercourse).

  V. Homosexual experiences (same as IV)

 VI. Group sex (same as IV)

VII. Marital experiences

   A. Sexual satisfaction in previous marriages; problems.

   B. Current marriage (beginnings of relationship, early sexual experiences; wedding night; honeymoon; differences before/after marriage; problems).

   C. Frequency of sexual activity in current marriage, desired frequency, quality changes desired, effects of drinking on sexual activity.

   D. Influences on sexual desire and frequency (who initiates; spontaneity; scheduled; habit; duty; time/place; degree of satisfaction with influences).

   E. Pregnancy History

   F. First noticed sexual problems, nature and extent of problems.

VIII. Extramarital sexual experiences (same as VII) including sex between marriages, widowhood, separation and divorce.

 IX. Feelings about self as sexual partner; male/female.

   A. For male and female: masculinity/femininity; sexual adequacy; acceptance of self; body image; genitalia; cross dressing.

  X. Sexual fantasies and dreams (nature and frequency); use of erotic materials.

 XI. Sexual deviations

   A. Homosexuality

   B. Sexual assault/incest/rape

   C. Voyeurism/exhibitionism/cross-dressing/fetishes/ transvestism

   D. Sadomasochism

   E. Prostitution

   F. Sexual contact with animals

XII. Effects of specific sexual activity
    A. Venereal disease (age, type, treatment, effects).
    B. Illegitimate pregnancies (same as A).
    C. Abortions
XIII. Sexual expectations in marriage, concept of effective sexual functioning.

APPLICATION TO AN ALCOHOLISM PROGRAM

It is the position of this paper that all alcoholism treatment should derive from the patient at least problem-oriented sexual information to determine if there is a problem, and its severity and impact on the recovery process. The minimal laboratory testing most programs should routinely conduct are prolactin, T^4 and serum testosterone levels. The questions listed are relevant to most stages of treatment:

Is there a problem?
What is the problem?
    What phase of the sexual response cycle is impaired?
    The nature and extent of the problem?
    How does the problem affect the individual? Couple?
What are its causes/etiology?
Are the sexual problems primary or secondary to a psychiatric problem?
What are the relationship issues relevant to the sexual problem?

The extent and intensity of the sexual problem history-taking will be determined by the skills of the clinicians doing the history, the patient's stability at the time, and the treatment setting itself. However, we are doing our alcoholic patients a disservice, in fact, we may be guilty of malpractice. if we do not at least ask basic questions about their sexual functioning. The recovery process of an alcoholic may be significantly impaired by sexual problems that never get addressed in treatment.

The detailed sex history can be utilized in total or in part by an alcoholism program, probably after a period of 3–6 months recovery. Unfortunately the greatest obstacle to good sexual history taking today appears to be the attitude and manner of alcoholism counselors themselves. Their anxiety and discomfort with the subject hampers the establishment of rapport and freedom of disclosure. Their own unresolved sexual attitudes and conflicts impede the patient interaction and impair their understanding of the patient's situation.

For example, unsuccessfully resolved homosexual anxiety may make it difficult for the counselor to frame questions on this subject, or to seek information about oral or anal sexual activity. The counselor that is convinced that the patient's sexual life is "none of his business" may be covering up unconscious anxiety and guilt feelings about intrusion to inhibit his questioning.

Therefore, it is imperative that alcoholism professionals receive further training in sexuality, and sex history-taking. If the alcoholism worker is truly interested in the alcoholic's general well-being and in maximizing the patient's potential for recovery, any understanding of the sexual impediments to treatment and sobriety is integral to the process. His responsibility to learn how to help alleviate suffering by improving sexual functioning seems inescapable.

BIBLIOGRAPHY

American Psychiatric Association. *Diagnostic and Statistical Manual III*. Washington, D.C. 1978.

Group for the Advancement of Psychiatry. *Assessment of Sexual Function: A Guide to Interviewing*. Vol. VIII. Report #88, January, 1977.

Hartman, William E., and Fithian, Marilyn A. *Treatment of Sexual Dysfunction: A Bio-Psycho-Social Approach*. Long Beach, CA.: Center for Marital and Sexual Studies, 1972.

Kaplan, Helen Singer. *The New Sex Therapy*. New York: Brunner/Mazel, 1974.

Kaplan, Helen Singer. *Disorders of Sexual Desire*. New York: Brunner/Mazel, 1979.

Kaplan, Helen Singer. *The Evaluation of Sexual Disorders*. New York: Brunner/Mazel, 1983.

Lief, Harold. "New Development in Sex Education of the Physician," *Journal of the American Medical Association*, 212, 1867–1986, 1970.

Masters, William, and Johnson, Virginia. *Human Sexual Inadequacy*. Boston: Little, Brown and Company, 1970.

Treatment of Impotence in Male Alcoholics

David J. Powell, Ph.D.

INTRODUCTION

Mr. John Smith has been admitted to Sobriety Hills, an alcoholism rehabilitation program. During intake, Mr. Smith's alcoholism counselor asks, "How's your sex life?" Mr. Smith responds, "Fine. Sure it could be better, but couldn't everything?" That's the last time the subject is raised, except for an entertaining and slightly uncomfortable lecture on "sex and booze" and a group therapy session on sex.

If the topic had been pursued it would have been found that Mr. Smith has a history of secondary impotence which has caused considerable anxiety and stress in the marriage. He bolsters his ego and courage with alcohol because of this anxiety to perform. Mrs. Smith has been anorgasmic for years. If tested, the rehabilitation program would have found that Mr. Smith has a low serum testosterone level (the hormone necessary for erection) and hyperprolactinemia (elevated prolactin levels). But the case is a success: Sobriety Hills has taught him to "stay out of bars," although they never addressed the subject of "what to do in bed."

Mr. Smith is an actual client who subsequently died from a tumor three years after leaving Sobriety Hills; he died sober. How common is Mr. Smith? The relationship between sexual problems and alcohol abuse had been well established. Clinical and laboratory research (Akhtar, 1977; Parades, 1975; Williams, 1976; Mendelson, 1974; Van Thiel, 1977; Lieber 1976; Gordon, 1979) supports Shakespeare's view that "alcohol provokes the desire, but takes away the performance." Research studies estimate from 40% (Kolodny, 1974) to 82% (Van Thiel, 1977) of male alcoholics experience impotence, as compared to 10% of the normal population. Although it is estimated that half of all males experience occasional transient episodes of impotence, that is within the limits of normal sexual behavior. However, alcohol-related impotence is a more severe or chronic form of this disorder.

Alcohol exerts multiple effects on the hypothalamic-pituitary-gonadal axis in alcoholic males (Kolodny, 1982). The effect on impotence is related to alcohol's damaging effect on the neurogenic reflex arc necessary for erection (Mallory, 1976; Lemere, 1973). Also associated sexual problems can result: gynecomastia, (enlargement of the breasts) atrophy of the testicles, inhibited sexual desire and sexual aversion (Todd, 1973). A significant number of alcoholic patients do experience impotence, rapid ejaculation and other sexual problems. All too often alcohologists treat just the alcohol problem. Although alcoholism counselors claim to treat the whole person, they rarely deal to any extent with the client's sexual and intimacy issues (Newman, 1976).

This paper will describe the nature of the problem, its etiology and incidence, various treatment approaches, and how to apply them to an alcoholism program. The paper will conclude with various training needs for the alcoholism specialist.

NATURE OF THE PROBLEM

Impotence occurs when the vascular reflex mechanism fails to pump sufficient blood into the cavernous sinuses of the penis to render it firm and erect. This may be due to physical and/or psychological factors (Masters, 1970).

Impotence can be divided into two clinical categories: primary impotent patients have never been potent with a partner, although some may attain good erections by masturbation or may experience nocturnal penile tumescence (NPT) and spontaneous erections in other situations. Secondary impotent patients have functioned well for some time prior to the development of their erectile dysfunction. In general, the prognosis is directly related to the symptom duration. Secondary impotence seems to have a more positive prognosis than primary impotence, which is more likely to be associated with serious psychological or neuroendocrine disorders (Kaplan, 1974).

Masters and Johnson (1970) indicate that alcoholism is the most prevalent factor for male secondary impotence for men in their 40s and 50s. Further, most alcoholics experiencing erectal dysfunction are secondarily impotent. Most alcoholics seem to have functioned well sexually for years. Once the alcoholism progresses into the dependency stage and the drinking pattern becomes more uniform, impotence is more pronounced.

Problems can also arise from drug treatment. Delayed ejaculation can be a side effect of treatment with Antabuse in approximately 16% of disulfiram users. Jensen showed that most alcoholic males experienced sexual dysfunction from their first day of Antabuse treatment but reported the same frequency of sexual activity. This finding indicates a shift in the qualitative experience of sexuality without necessarily a quantitative change.

Based on laboratory research (Lemere, 1973; Van Thiel, 1977), the organic etiology for impotent alcoholics is significantly higher than 15% (the figure used by Masters and Johnson for the degree of organicity in impotent males). This is due to the direct effect of alcohol on the sex steroids and the gonadotropins: decreased production of testosterone, a relative or absolute shift towards greater estrogenicity, impaired sperm production, increased hepatic 5 testosterone-reductase (which serves to break down testosterone), alterations in the central regulatory balance mechanisms (Luteinizing hormone/Follicule stimulating hormone) an increased percentage of testosterone bound to protein and elevated prolactin levels. Prolactin may modulate the level of estrogen receptors in the liver Luteinizing hormone receptors in the testes. Further, alcoholic polyneuropathy is a well-established complication of chronic alcoholism, mainly affecting the somatic peripheral nerves (Bjork, 1977).

Many patients in an alcoholic marriage experience a full range of associated psychological and relationship issues: lack of trust, communication breakdowns, control and power struggles, feelings of isolation and depression, loss of self-esteem, blurred sexual identity, and feelings of hostility and anxiety. All of these may contribute to the psychological etiology of impotence.

ETIOLOGY

Chinese physicians from 1000 B.C. wrote that masturbation induced impotence (as well as insanity and blindness). Throughout history a variety of causative factors were postulated for impotence. Hippocrates noted in 400 B.C that a "preoccupation with male affairs and a lack of womanly attractiveness" were causative factors behind impotence. In the Bible (Genesis 20:1), erectile failure was believed to be the result of a divine curse. Even as recent as the

1800s, Dr. Benjamin Rush noted that "undue or a promiscuous intercourse with the female sex . . . produces seminal weakness, impotence." Freud held that disgust resulting from a child's discovery that his mother had no penis could produce impotence.

Other psychological factors have been postulated: coital anxiety, fear of failure or ridicule, fear of inflicting injury on the partner, "vagina dentata" theory (wherein the male fantasizes that the vaginal orifice acts as a mouth with teeth), hostility and resentment, and undue sensitivity to criticism. Kinsey suggested that ignorance of the normal biological variation in sexual performance was associated with impaired potency; for example, some people believe "a drop of semen is equal to a pint of blood." The 1945 U.S. Boy Scout Manual warned youth against "wasting their vital fluid for fear it would be all expended." Other patterns of erectile problems can be related to fear of discovery, pregnancy or guilt. In these cases, erectile problems result after vaginal penetration but prior to ejaculation. Masters and Johnson (1981) have postulated a 10–15% physiological basis for impotence. Kaplan (1974) reiterated this assertion by stating that 85% of impotence is psychogenic. However, she also commented that impotent males are "burdened by an especially reactive vasocongestive genital system" in general.

The complex hormonal, vascular, and neural mechanisms that mediate erection are also vulnerable to physical agents like alcohol. Therefore, unless the erectile difficulty is clearly situational, the physiological and anatomical integrity of these mechanisms should be explored. Associated physical causes should be diagnosed: stress, fatigue, diabetes, low androgen levels, hepatic problems, estrogenic and parasympatholytic medication, neurological diseases, tumors, multiple sclerosis, Peyronie's disease of the penis, urological problems, etc. All of these associated physical problems can be found in frequent numbers in male alcoholic populations. Therefore, the physiological basis for alcoholic impotence is clear and must be diagnosed and explored by alcohologists in treatment programs.

Clinical practice has shown more immediate operating factors as the etiology of impotence: performance anxiety is the most frequent psychological cause of the problem. Many men experience some form of impaired erectile capacity at times in their sexual lives. For most, it is situational and can be dismissed as normal. However, for some it becomes a reflection on their masculinity or manhood. When impotence occurs, conscious or unconscious performance anxiety precedes it and emotional devastation follows. When a man has unpredictable episodes of impotence, his sexual life becomes colored by fear and anxiety (Kaplan, 1974).

Most men demand that their sexual performance be perfect at all times. Although it is understandable that the best baseball players rarely bat above .300 and the best golfers still have bogeys, sexual activity demands higher standards of performance. That is performance anxiety.

This anxiety can have origins in another problem: rapid ejaculation. Often when you see an impotent male, you are also probably seeing a male who has had problems with ejaculation (Masters, 1982). He becomes anxious that he will ejaculate too quickly, so tries everything possible, thinking terrible, morbid thoughts, distractions, and even muscular desensitization. If he is really good at it, he will deaden the system entirely and eventually become impotent. It works; he needn't worry about disappointing his partner by ejaculating too soon. Of course, impotence brings other more complex problems. To summarize, impotence can have both physiological and psychological origins. In the alcoholic male it is likely that both factors are involved.

TREATMENT APPROACHES

The first step in treating impotent males is to take a thorough history. To clarify the differential diagnosis of psychogenic and organic origins. Table I outlines a plan of medical examination of the patient. A detailed verbal sex history should also be taken (Powell, "Sex History-Taking and the Alcoholism Worker"). Of course, not all of the tests in Table I are needed all the time. They are listed to indicate the intensity of testing that may be necessary.

The next task is to subdivide the patients into primary and secondary cases (Table II) including "sometimes" and "always" present. The duration, development, and degree of erectile dysfunction should be thoroughly elucidated, including rigidity of morning erections; nocturnal penile tumescence; and whether the failure exists in all positions, with different heterosexual and homosexual partners, or with masturbation. Immediate causative issues need to be explored: smoking habits, medications, drug abuse, etc. A full physical examination should be given.

TABLE I: A PLAN FOR MEDICAL EXAMINATION OF MALE IMPOTENCE

General:
  Detail sex history
  Physical status/anatomic conditions (including vascular status)
  Neurolocal and endocrine conditions (impaired sensory pathways, chronic pain, impaired sexual reflexes, adrenal disorders, hypogonadism, thyroid disorders, pituitary disorders)
  Other conditions (liver disease, malignancy, infections in the pelvic region, kidney disease, urologic disorders)

Diagnostic Testing:

  Complete physical examination
  Clinical laboratory testing (CBC, Urinalysis, VDRL, g.c. cultures, chemistry screening profiles, serum testosterone, LH/FSH, prolactin, T^4, glucose tolerance test)
  Genital reflexes (cystometry)
  Stimulation plethysmography (visual/vibration)
  Penile blood pressure (rest/postocclusive)
  Penile pulse amplitude (Doppler)
  Nocturnal plethysmography (NPT)
  Invasive factors (blood flow, infusion cavernosography, arteriography)

TABLE II: TYPES OF ERECTILE PROBLEMS
(Graber, 1979)

TYPE	CRITERIA
Erectile problems with intercourse, primary and always	Never been functional in intercourse: continuous history
Problems primary and sometimes	Generally had a history of erectile problems; occasionally functional; never free of anxiety of problem

To illustrate the need for a physical exam, the following case example is presented:

A client was diagnosed as impotent for psychogenic reasons: fear of painful intercourse. No physical or neuroendocrine basis was found upon examination. The treatment was unsuccessful until an examination was conducted wherein a penile plethysmography test was used in an erect state. The examination revealed a narrow slit at the base of the coronal ridge which caused considerable pain when he was erect. This cut was imperceptible in the flaccid state. Thus, the patient had conditioned himself to be impotent for fear of pain upon erection. The pain, however, was initially assumed to be associated with intercourse and insertion, since he was examined in the flaccid state.

Once a physiological etiology has been established, treatment may involve the following approaches: hormone supplementation (Afrodex), testosterone treatment, corrective surgery on the arterial supply or on drainage failures, and prosthetic implant surgery. However, according to Masters and Johnson (1982), a significant number (50%) of impotence cases with organic etiology respond successfully to psychotherapy. Therefore, whatever the etiology, treatment of erectile dysfunction should probably involve psychotherapy.

A number of basic sex therapy principles apply in psychotherapy for erectile problems:

1. Establishment of a climate of effective interaction via:
   a. neutrality—staying in the present
   b. acceptance—not assigning blame for feelings of self or the partner
   c. responsibility for self—"I am not responsible for my feelings, only my actions." Uncomfortable feelings are dealt with by acting to help oneself rather than by analyzing the feelings or depending on the partner to correct the feelings.
2. Building communication skills:
   a. being aware of thoughts, perceptions, feelings and desires
   b. developing adequate vocabulary to communicate feelings
   c. overcoming defenses
   d. self-representation, "I" messages
   e. negotiation, giving priority to the best interests of the relationship, taking into account whose needs are the greatest
   f. brainstorming and problem solving skills

g. dealing with manipulations

h. development of listening skills

Another principle is that "there is no such entity as an uninvolved partner in a marriage contending with any form of sexual dysfunction" (Masters, 1970). Impotence is a unit or relationship problem and not the male's issue solely. Therefore, whenever possible, the male and female should be treated simultaneously.

Further, Masters and Johnson (1970) state that the secret of successful therapy for impotence is not to treat the symptom of impotence. Erection is a natural process and isolating the symptom is to try to will something natural. The client should realize that he need not learn to have an erection: it will happen just as voluntarily as breathing if the other physiological and psychological factors are intact. Thus, the roadblocks to potency must be addressed: performance anxiety, fear of failure and vulnerability to emotional arousal. The three main goals of psychotherapy for impotence are to remove the fears of performance, reeducate the patient to being a participant and not spectator to the sexual process, and relieve the partner's fears about the man's sexual activities. To accomplish these goals, a brief, symptom-focussed behaviorally-oriented form of therapy seems to work better than lengthy, reconstructive, insight-oriented therapy.

To reduce fears of performance and vulnerability to emotional arousal, clients are taught to remove or avoid stressful situations, i.e., to resist all demands for sex. To help this process, intercourse is usually restricted. Restoration of confidence is critical to treatment; therefore, we seek to enhance the stimulating factors and diminished those that engender anxiety.

Besides eliminating intercourse temporarily, treatment begins with a period of ejaculatory abstinence and non-erectile oriented, teasing, erotic stimulation (Kaplan, 1974). When erectile confidence is restored, coitus is resumed. The specific therapeutic approaches follow.

1. An educational process that sex is a natural psychophysiological function.

2. Removal of blocks like misinformation and lack of knowledge about anatomy and physiology. For example, a patient could not understand how his wife urinated with a tampon inserted. Since he feared hurting her urinary functions with inter-

course, impotence seemed the best alternative. A brief "guided tour" by his wife of her sexual anatomy quickly alleviated this fear and misinformation.

3. Non-demand pleasuring involving touching of the non-genital and subsequently, genital areas. The emphasis is not on sexual performance but on mutual enhancement of non-orgasmic erotic pleasures. Erection and arousal are not expected. Teasing, spontaneous erections occur during these pleasuring sessions. The couple learns that erections can occur spontaneously when not impaired by pressure and anxiety.

4. Dispelling the fear of failure. This can be accomplished by teaching the squeeze technique to dispel the anxiety and fear of failure. (The squeeze technique involves placing the female's thumb on the interior surface of the penis and the first and second fingers at the superior/exterior penis surface immediately adjacent to one another on either side of the coronal ridge. Pressure is applied by squeezing steadily the thumb and two fingers together for three to four seconds. This should immediately result in the loss of urge to ejaculate (Masters, 1970). (See Figure 1.) Another experiential tactic to be used to dispel the fear of failure: systematic fondling of the penis, interrupted temporarily to allow the erection to abate (Nowinski).

5. Distracting obsessive thoughts. Some patients still are obsessed with questions: "Will I get an erection?" "Will I lose it?" "Is this really going to work long-term?" Distraction can be taught by focussing on erotic sensations, thought-stopping, desensitization, muscular relaxation, or detachment from the ongoing situation via fantasy. For some, the obsessive thoughts are deeply rooted in the unconscious sources which must be dealt with before the thoughts cease.

6. Permission-giving to be "selfish." "Is she going to climax?" "Is she enjoying this?" "Am I a good lover?" These fears foster spectatoring wherein the male mentally steps outside the process and watches himself "doing it." He denies himself potential biophysical input by spectatoring. In sex therapy for impotence, the male is taught to be temporarily selfish, to focus on his own sexual gratification.

When asked what makes a good lover, most men will respond, "The ability to stay erect for hours, and to give your

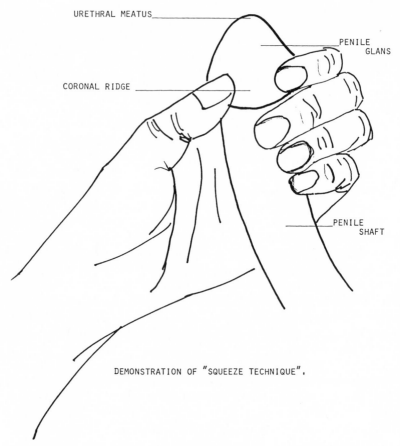

URETHRAL MEATUS

PENILE GLANS

CORONAL RIDGE

PENILE SHAFT

DEMONSTRATION OF "SQUEEZE TECHNIQUE".

FIGURE 1

partner multiple orgasms." However, sexual enjoyment is found to a large extent in the person's ability to abandon himself to his erotic or sensual feelings and to thoroughly enjoy himself, still being sensitive to his partner's needs and pleasures. In this case, selfishness does not mean disregard of the partner's needs, but exquisite sensitivity and mutual generosity. The principle of "taking turns" is taught to free the person from the obsession with solely pleasuring himself or his partner to the exclusion of the other. Sensate focus exercises aid in this learning process.

7. After confidence has returned, coitus may be resumed via mu-

tual pleasuring with the female in the astride position. The female, in a heterosexual relationship, is given charge to insert the penis when she desires and to gently move her hips in a rhythmic, non-demanding manner. Initially, ejaculation should occur after they separate. Extravaginal penile stimulation is encouraged as well as erotic fantasies.

In sex therapy practice, the husband in an alcoholic marriage does not solely bear the onus for the difficulties. The wife may place a variety of obstacles in the way. She may still be carrying excessive resentment and anger. She may refuse to let him "get well." "After all he has done to me, he is going to pay a little." The wife may create tension and a quarrelsome environment to strike back at his progress. She may sabotage the process by complaining about his performance. She may be "hedging her bet" by silently saying, "Bet you can't give me an orgasm." The partner may be invested in the symptomatology. "See how sick he is." She may play the spectator role and thus heighten his anxiety to perform. She may unconsciously be fearful of his recovery. "If he becomes potent, it will be clear that I am dysfunctional too. Let's keep the focus off me and on him" (Masters, 1982).

To treat these issues, Alanon's principle of detachment is appropriate. The wife's anger and resentment must be dealt with; her sabotaging of the process should be confronted in a supportive manner. Her role in the dysfunction needs to be addressed as well as her fears of failure or success. The partner's attitudes about himself, her, sex, and the relationship should be dealt with as well as the emotions associated with the impotence (rejection, frustration, blame). She should be given permission to be sexual again by providing information related to female sexuality and emphasizing responsibility for her own sexual expression. The feelings of learned helplessness need to be confronted. Without modifying these problems, the therapy may continuously be sabotaged by the wife.

APPLICATION TO ALCOHOLISM TREATMENT PROGRAMS

In a recent conversation with Dr. William Masters (1982) he stated, "Alcohologists are guilty of malpractice if they do not adequately explore the organic etiology of sexual problems." Problems such as low serum testosterone levels may involve hyperprolac-tinemia (elevated prolactin levels) which may result in blindness and facial tumors. Alcoholic clients like Mr. Smith in the introduction may be dying of brain tumors after years of sobriety because no one made the connection to the sexual dysfunctions.

Most counselors will acknowledge the relationship between drinking and sexual problems. Most will even state that these problems need to be treated at some time. However, that is as far as many alcohologists go, except for a tacit acknowledgement of the problem via a lecture on sexuality or a group therapy discussion. What can be done in a 28-day rehabilitation program? We can't treat everything. First things first; sobriety is paramount! Besides, in the aftercare community, most people treating sexual problems don't understand the needs of the alcoholic. So goes the litany in the alcoholism field.

What can be done? If we acknowledge the importance of the sexual issues and possibly even the life threatening potential of the problems, we then need to look for ways to incorporate sexual issues into our programs. The first step is to demystify sex therapy. For years, alcoholism counselors put family therapy in a separate category. "We cannot deal with the family. It is an aftercare issue. We have no expertise in family therapy." Once the importance of the family was accepted by alcohologists, we learned about family therapy. We hired family specialists. We incorporated the family into the treatment plan.

The alcoholism community has the same hesitancy with sex therapy. There is a mystique that sex therapy is a higher order, more complex form of counseling. Yet when one looks at the above section on the principles of sex therapy, clearly there are strong parallels to alcoholism counseling in general:

1. Sex therapy uses the concept that sexual problems are unit problems, even as we say alcoholism is a family disease.
2. Both are reality based, dealing for the most part with the "here and now."
3. Both are behavioral in nature, using specific principles to change behaviors.
4. Both involve client education.
5. Both deal with the partner's resentments and anger via detachment.

6. Both teach problem-solving, negotiation, communication and listening skills.

Sex therapy involves counseling an individual or relationship about intimacy and sexual issues. Some alcoholism counselors may border on doing sex counseling and not realize it. When they treat the individual with concerns for closeness, affection, communication and intimacy issues, they are not far from doing counseling. This is not to imply that there is not a specific body of knowledge and skills involved in sex therapy. It does not mean that every alcoholism counselor can title himself a sex therapist because he deals with intimacy issues. It does mean that sex therapy needs to be seen as a separate but integral component of individual and couple counseling. It is certainly within the realm of most alcoholism treatment programs.

What can be done in a rehabilitation program? At a minimum upon intake the program should conduct routine laboratory work-ups on serum testosterone levels, and if indicated, prolactin and T^4 levels. The cost to an Alcohol Rehabilitation Unit is minimal; the benefit is to screen out organicity in sexual problems that may interfere with the client's sexual functioning. If he has a fatty liver, we will want to tell him that. If he has neuroendocrine problems that may interfere with his sexual life we should inform the client of that also.

However, just deriving that information and sharing it with the client is not sufficient and may, in fact, be destructive to the rehabilitation without further incorporation of treatment approaches into the rehabilitation process. An adaptation of the PLISSIT (Annon) model can be utilized to incorporate sexual counseling into an alcoholism program. PLISSIT is a simplified, minimal approach to dealing with sexual problems in alcoholics, an approach that could be adopted by most residential and aftercare treatment programs.

PLISSIT stand for: P—Permission giving
  LI—Limited Information
  SS—Specific Suggestions
  IT—Intensive Therapy

This model is adaptable to the degree of client contact, treatment goals and clinician skill levels. Each level involves greater degrees of clinical sophistication, training and knowledge.

PERMISSION-GIVING

As the haze clears in the recovering alcoholic's mind, questions often occur regarding sexual performance. They wonder if there is something wrong with them, are they abnormal because they experienced sexual problems. In Permission-Giving, the clinician assures them they are not alone; it is only natural that they would experience some problems after years of drinking. This simple reassurance can reduce performance anxiety and resolve some of the simpler problems.

Also, Permission-Giving establishes an open climate for discussion and sharing of feelings, thoughts, fantasies, dreams, and behaviors. The counselor communicates his/her comfort level in discussing sexual issues and says to the client, "I'm willing to talk about it when you are." Covert concerns and overt behaviors are open topics of discussion. Often Permission-Giving is sufficient to stop recurring sexual obsessions associated with anxiety about potency.

The Client can be given permission *not* to engage in certain sexual behaviors unless they choose to. They need not feel the pressure to perform sexually immediately after treatment. The impotent alcoholic male does not have to subject himself to erectile performance at this stage of recovery.

This does not mean the clinician gives "blanket" permission to engage or not engage in any type of sexual behaviors. Adverse consequences of behaviors need to be pointed out. Legal considerations need to be clear, especially regarding sexual activity with children, rape, etc.

Permission-Giving can occur in an alcoholism treatment unit in a number of ways:

1. An introductory statement can be given by the clinician from the onset of treatment that sexual issues can be discussed freely. This is done through opening statements, questions on the intake about sexual issues, comments about sexuality and alcoholism early on in treatment, etc.
2. Make literature on sexuality and alcoholism available at the unit library, on the ward, etc.
3. Display posters at the center about sexual performance. A number of eye-catching posters are available from the Addi-

tions Research Foundation of Ontario, Canada, and United States groups.

All of these techniques convey an openness about sexuality and give permission to the clients to discuss sexual problems in greater depth.

LIMITED INFORMATION

Limited Information provides the client specific factual data directly relevant to his particular sexual concerns. For example, an alcoholic client was very anxious about sex because his penis was "too small" (4½ inches by his measurement). He had read that the average penis was six inches. The client was provided simple factual information about average flaccid vs. erect penis size, the average length of the female vagina (3–4"), the sparsity of nerve endings inside the vagina, etc. This simple information was sufficient to reduce the client's concerns and anxieties.

The common areas of individual concerns center around myths about breast and genital size, sexual interest/appetite, responsiveness, orgasmic potential, masturbation, oral-genital contact, sexual frequency, etc. However, research has indicated that three hours of broad sexual information has little direct influence on changing a client's problems. For example, it is not very useful to have a general lecture on intimacy and sexuality for an alcoholic population unless specific information about sexual dysfunction and alcoholism is provided. The gain from such a lecture is more in the area of permission-giving and setting a climate for discussion that in changing specific attitudes and behaviors. In an alcoholism treatment unit, the Limited Information should be focussed on the alcoholics' concern for impotence, rapid ejaculation, anorgasmia, and inhibited sexual desire, many of which occur in the sexual life of the alcoholic couple. This can be done via:

1. A presentation on specific sexual dysfunctions and alcoholism,
2. Structured group therapy discussions on sexual problems,
3. Individual counseling sessions aimed at each client's specific needs and

4. Couple/family counseling sessions dealing with intimacy/sexuality.

SPECIFIC SUGGESTIONS

Limited Information is usually as far as an alcoholism treatment program goes in dealing with sexual issues. This is primarily because before clinicians can give detailed, specific suggestions to the client, they first need information about the client's sexual history. Here is where the field divides. Most say, and probably rightly so, that we don't have time in a twenty-eight day program to do a detailed sex history. When you start to take a comprehensive sex history you are heading into intensive therapy. However, there is time to take a sexual problem history, focussing on the items in Table III. Additionally, the medical information in Table I becomes part of the sexual problem history. A sexual problem history can be easily adapted to a ten minute or one hour format. It forms the basis for the Specific Suggestions.

In Permission-Giving and Limited Information the clinician does most of the work. In Specific Suggestions, the client must take active steps to change his/her behaviors and attitudes within a brief therapy framework typical of most alcoholism treatment units.

Annon (1975) begins with two sayings that form the context for Specific Suggestions: (1) "It is what you do with what you have, rather than what you have that counts." (2) "There is always another time." These sayings are principles that are given to the alcoholic client to reduce anxiety and to build a repertoire of thought-stopping devices when stress occurs. Specific Suggestions are targeted to each individual client's needs, and typically involve for the alcoholic male: redirection of attention, thought-stopping techniques; muscular relaxation and systematic desensitization; graded sexual responses ("You don't always have a seven course meal; sometimes just a snack."); sensate focus techniques; negotiation skills; interrupted stimulation; squeeze techniques; and genital muscle training (Kegel's). These suggestions are of three types for the impotent male: Male oriented only, female partner oriented only, and couple oriented.

The alcoholism counselor may also give the client specific readings as a means to provide Limited Information and Specific Suggestions. Examples of readings may be Nowinski, *Becoming Satisfied* and *The Great Orgasm Robbery*; Weinberg, *Sex and Recovery*;

or Raley, *Making Love*. To aid the male in better understanding female sexuality, readings such as Barbach, *For Yourself* and LoPiccolo, *Becoming Orgasmic*, can be suggested. However, there is a danger in using readings: they can become an easy escape for the clinician from having to deal with the client's individual needs. They can also be inappropriately suggested to certain clients. It is essential that every reading recommended be based on familiarity with the client's needs and reactions to sexually explicit material.

An Alcoholism Treatment Unit library should contain the above readings as well as other articles and books on sexuality and alcoholism. Further, upon intake and throughout the counseling process, the clinician should elicit sexual problem history information and incorporate it into the client's treatment plan. Specific suggestions can become part of the ongoing therapy as issues recycle. Rather than separate sexual counseling from the rest of the treatment program, sex should be included as part of all aspects of the counseling. Upon discharge the client should be given the names of sex counselors for those in need of further therapy in the aftercare community.

INTENSIVE THERAPY

Based upon the limited sexual problem history taken, the clinician should determine the degree of pathology and the need for more intensive therapy. It is beyond the scope of most residential rehabilitation programs to do intensive sex therapy while in-patient. However, intensive therapy should be offered as part of the aftercare plan for clients with serious sexual problems.

How does an Alcoholism Treatment Unit find a competent sex therapist? The American Association of Sex Educators, Counselors, and Therapists (AASECT) has certification standards for counselors and therapists and can be consulted about people that meet these standards. However, further study of the sex therapists; familiarity with substance abuse is necessary for an appropriate referral for a recovering alcoholic. Each treatment program should develop a list of sex therapists in the community who can deal with alcoholic couples/clients, just as referral lists are kept for family therapists, physicians, criminal justice system personnel, etc.

Most of the above has been focussed on the residential alcoholism program. For the out-patient clinician or agency, all aspects of the PLISSIT model can be incorporated into treatment. Group lectures and therapy sessions can include Permission-Giving, Limited Information and Specific Suggestions. Ongoing intensive therapy can be provided as part of individual, group and couple therapy. When should sexual issues be brought into the out-patient treatment program? The basic principle for sexual counseling (and for that matter, for any area of counseling) is that nothing should be done that jeopardizes the precarious sobriety of the alcoholic. Beyond this rule, however, sexual issues should be addressed from the onset of treatment, working gradually through the PLISSIT steps. Typically, intensive therapy does not begin for the alcoholic couple until an initial stable period (six months) of sobriety has been established.

TRAINING NEEDS

The recommended principle is: If you aren't one, become one. There is no reason why the alcoholism counselor cannot get basic training in the treatment of problems with sexuality, intimacy, sexual dysfunctions, treatment approaches, etc. Workshops, conferences and training programs are available throughout the United States that provide introductions to the subjects. Every alcoholism counselor should have basic training in sex counseling and alcoholism treatment programs should seek to hire these personnel as counselors on their staff.

A number of training programs are available in the alcoholism field that provide a good introductory background and workshops are available through AASECT, colleges and universities, American Association of Marriage and Family Therapy, Masters and Johnson Institute, etc.

The most critical ethical issues, though, is that alcoholism counselors should not profess to be sex counselors without appropriate training and credentialling. Don't say you are when you aren't. Perhaps more so than any other area of counseling, sexual issues need to be dealt with appropriately and ethically.

CONCLUSION

To continue to avoid sexual issues for the alcoholic is to do the client a disservice and is unprofessional for the field. It is time that the alcohologist incorporates all factors when treating the whole

person and treatment of sexuality/sexual dysfunctions are critical to
the recovery process.

BIBLIOGRAPHY

Akhtar, M.M. "Sexual Disorders in Male Alcoholics," in W. Madden (ed.) *Alcoholism and Drug Dependence*. N.Y.: Plenum Press, 1977.

Annon, J.S. *The Behavioral Treatment of Sexual Problems*, Vol. 2. Honolulu: Enabling Systems, 1975.

Barbach, L. *For Yourself: The Fulfillment of Female Sexuality*. N.Y.: Anchor Press, 1975.

Bjork, J.T. "Clomiphene Citrate Therapy in a Patient with Laennec's Cirrhosis", *Gastroenterology*, 72(6): 1308–11, 1977.

Gordon, G.G., Southren, A.L., Vittek, J., and Lieber, C.S. "The Effect of Alcohol Ingestion on Hepatic Aromatese Activity and Plasma Steroid Hormones," *Metabolism*. N.Y. 28:20–24, 1979.

Graber, G. and Graber, B. *Woman's Orgasm*. Indianapolis: Bobbs-Merrill, 1975.

Kaplan, H.S. *The New Sex Therapy: Active Treatment Of Sexual Dysfunction*. N.Y.: Brunner/Mazel, 1974.

Kolodny, R.C., Masters, W.H., Kolodner, R.M. and Toro, G. "Depression of Plasma Testosterone Levels After Chronic Intensive Marijuana Use", *New England Journal of Medicine* Vol. 290:872–874, 1974.

Kolodny, R.C. Post Graduate Seminar on Human Sexual Dysfunction. St. Louis, Missouri. 1982.

Lemere, F. and Smith, M.W. "Alcohol-Induced Sexual Impotence", *American Journal of Psychiatry*, 130(2): 212–3, 1973.

LoPiccolo, L., Heimen, J., and LoPiccolo, J. *Becoming Orgasmic: A Sexual Growth Program for Women*. Englewood Cliffs, N.J.: Prentice-Hall, 1976.

Mallory, E.S. "Strategies in Sexual Counseling In Alcoholic Marriage", In: Joseph Newman, *Sexual Counseling For Persons With Alcohol Problems*. U. of Pittsburgh, 1976.

Masters, W.H. Personal Conversation, St. Louis, Missouri, 1981.

Masters, W.H. and Johnson, V.E. *Human Sexual Inadequacy*. Boston: Little, Brown, 1970.

Masters, W.H. and Johnson, V.E. Post Graduate Seminar on Human Sexual Dysfunction. St. Louis, Missouri, 1982.

Mendelson, J. and Mello, N. "Alcohol, Aggression and Androgens", *Aggression*. 52:225–47, 1974.

Newman, J. *Sexual Counseling for Persons with Alcohol Problems*. U. of Pittsburgh, 1976.

Nowinski, J. *Becoming Satisfied*. Englewood Cliffs, N.J.: Prentice-Hall, 1980.

Parades, A. "Marital-Sexual Factors in Alcoholism", unpublished paper. Oklahoma City, Oklahoma, 1975.

Powell, D.J. "Sexual Dysfunction & Alcoholism", *Journal of Sex Education & Therapy*, 6(2): 40–46, 1980.

Powell, D.J. "Sex History Taking In Alcoholism", unpublished paper, 1980.

Rubin, W. and Leiber, C. *Information and Feature Service*. Washington, D.C.: NIAAA, 1976.

Todd, W.H. "Truth About Sex and Alcohol", *Memorial Mercury*. 13(4): 15–6, 1973.

Van Thiel, D.H., Gaveler, Judith S., and Lester, R. "Tehanol: A Gonadal Toxin in the Female", *Drug and Alcohol Dependence*. 2(5/6): 373–80, 1977.

Van Thiel, D. "Testicular and Spermatozoal Auto-Antibody in Chronic Alcoholics with Gonadal Failure", *Clinical Immunology and Immunopathology*. 8:311–7, 1977.

Weinberg, J. *Sex & Recovery*. Minneapolis: Recovery Press, 1977.

Williams, K. "Overview of Sexual Problems in Alcoholism", In: Joseph Newman, *Sexual Counseling for Persons with Alcohol Problems*. U. of Pittsburgh, 1976.

Special Issues Affecting the Treatment of Gay Male and Lesbian Alcoholics

Gay

Dana G. Finnegan, Ph.D.
David Cook, C.S.W.

Approximately ten percent of the general population is homosexual (Kinsey, Pomeroy, Martin, 1948; Kinsey, Pomeroy, Martin and Gebhart, 1953). Since Kinsey's studies, no one has seriously challenged that statistic. Accordingly, if people counsel alcoholics, they are bound to counsel some who are also gay males or lesbians. And since alcoholism counselors are certain to be counseling some gay and lesbian clients, it is imperative that counselors realize that these clients are subject to the same sexual issues, problems, dysfunctions, and anxieties as straight clients. It is even more important, however, for counselors to realize that their gay and lesbian clients must deal with some very special issues and problems in addition to the ones that all alcoholics face. The primary issues which increase the burden of the gay/lesbian alcoholic struggling to recover are homophobia (the irrational fear of homosexuality), both external and internalized homophobia and intensified defensive reactions (e.g., heightened denial).

In order to treat their gay and lesbian clients in constructive and health-enhancing ways, counselors must be able to determine when to focus on their clients' alcoholism and basically ignore their sexual orientation and when to attend closely to client's sexual orientation and the interplay between it and the alcoholism. Although the counselor needs always to be sensitive to sexual orientation, there are times when it must be directly addressed if it is creating problems for the client. Being able to make such determinations accurately and somewhat objectively and being able to carry out the treatment in a sensitive manner requires that counselors have significantly tempered their own homophobia and that they have acquired a fair amount of knowledge of gay/lesbian lifestyles. Being able to do this also requires that counselors have a repertoire of methods which directly address the issues particular to gay/lesbian alcohol-

© 1984 by The Haworth Press, Inc. All rights reserved.

85

ics' recovery processes. In effect, counselors need to know some specific "how-to's".

This article will focus on three basic areas of concern: the particular issues which may make recovery harder for gay/lesbian alcoholics; the relationship of these issues to treatment; and some practical suggestions for counselors.

The central issues from which all other issues spring and without which gay and lesbian alcoholics would be just simple alcoholics is homophobia; the intense, irrational fear of homosexuality and homosexuals (Weinberg, 1972). Since being coined by Weinberg, this term has broadened to include disgust, contempt, and rage towards homosexuality and now denotes any negative feeling toward homosexuality.

Because homophobia is embedded in the very bones of our culture, probably no one in this society completely escapes being socialized to be homophobic. Society's anti-homosexual attitudes and teachings constitute external homophobia; that which is imposed on the individual primarily by four societal institutions.

Citing chapters from Leviticus and elsewhere, religions have led the attack on homosexuality, claiming that it strikes at the very heart of what Judeo-Christian cultures value most: marriage and family. Thus most religions have branded homosexuality as wicked, sinful, immoral, and against the laws of God and Nature. Unfortunately, the virulence of these claims has not noticeably lessened over the years, and, in fact, from time to time ministers from some of the less restrained religious groups call for the suppression and sometimes the extermination of homosexuals. Perhaps the most current example of homophobia with strong religious overtones is the contention that homosexual males who have AIDS deserve what they get; that like the inhabitants of Sodom and Gomorrah, they are being punished for their sins.

The late 1800s saw the development of another point of view. The medical profession turned its attention to homosexuality and concluded that it was a sickness, an aberration, an abnormality. While the newer theoretical perspective did not replace the religious view, it did temper it somewhat. Basically, two etiologies were posited. One was that homosexuality is caused by hormonal imbalances or deficits. The other psychoanalytic view was that homosexuality resulted from sexual immaturity. One example of this view was that homosexual boys are created by having a "close binding mother" and a "distant or absent" father (Bieber et al., 1962). Although neither theory is supported by evidence (Myers, 1982) and although the American Psychiatric Association voted in 1973 to remove homosexuality as an illness from its diagnostic manual, much of the medical and psychological profession continues to view and to treat homosexuals as sick people who need to be "cured" (American Psychiatric Association, 1980; Knutson, 1980).

The third major institution which supports homophobia is the law. Since the function of law is to enforce the beliefs and values of society, it is not surprising that homosexual behavior between consenting adults is still illegal and punishable by jail terms in twenty-nine states (Vetri, 1980). Oppression by omission is equally powerful. In most cities and states, homosexuals are not clearly protected by civil rights laws. In New York City, for example, a ten-year battle to grant civil rights specifically to gays has been defeated each year by factions led by Catholics and Orthodox Jews. Without such protection, homosexuals can be and frequently are discriminated against. They can be refused housing, evicted, and fired without recourse under the law.

The fourth institution which perpetuates and reinforces external homophobia is the media. Direct statements about homosexuality as a deficiency, a disease, and a sin appear with distressing frequency in columns of newspapers across the country. What little television coverage is given of gay/lesbian activities sometimes presents a rather negative view (e.g., *60 Minutes'* presentation on "Gay Politics, Gay Power" in San Francisco). When television shows have gay or lesbian characters, they are usually silly and inconsequential at best, or they are presented as tragic creatures. Although there are certainly exceptions to all of these instances, the majority of media presentations are either subtly or blatantly homophobic. In addition, much homophobia is conveyed by omission. Any random, even casual, examination of television programs reveals that they do not present homosexual characters often, and only rarely do they present an admirable homosexual character, one who might serve as a role model for those viewers who are themselves homosexual or as an example of a healthy homosexual for those viewers who are heterosexual. What occurs is shaped by "heterosexism," the assumption that everyone is heterosexual (except for a few unfortunates) and that anyone who is not heterosexual would really rather be so if only that were possible.

If gays and lesbians had only to contend with the homophobia in society, that would be hard enough. But the cruelest irony is that homophobia does not stay only out there in society. As children born and raised primarily by heterosexual parents in a homophobic culture, gay men and lesbians learn by osmosis to be homophobic. They internalize the homophobia which permeates society and thereby learn to fear and hate that which makes up their identity and which constitutes the very core of their being: not just their sexual orientation, but their very "way of being in the world." This core becomes their enemy so that now they have two hostile and rejecting enemies: one that is outside, one that is within.

Internalized homophobia takes many forms and has many effects, some subtle, some blatant. People who have it learn to think, feel, and act in response to their internalized homophobia. Often they think that people who are straight are superior, that gays (including themselves) are inferior. They may think that even though they are gay they should marry, have children, and live a heterosexual life style because to be gay is sinful or unnatural. They may even learn to think of themselves as not-gay, as straight, because to think any other way is too painful or too frightening. Hatred, loathing, contempt, fear: these and many other negative feelings crowd the souls of many homosexuals. The feelings generated by internalized homophobia have wide-ranging and often very negative ramifications for gays and lesbians. Self-hatred and self-loathing are destructive to ego development and functioning; they can contribute to depression, suicidal thoughts or behavior, alcoholism, drug abuse, and addictions of whatever type. These feelings often serve to cut one gay person off from another. (Since gayness is so horrible, I hate it in me and in anyone else.) Isolation and mistrust are often the result.

Fear, deep and powerful, is also created by internalized homophobia. If what comprises the core of one's being is believed to be contemptible and immoral, there is a fear of discovery by others. (What would they think of me if they only knew?) Another fear is that of discovery by self. (Maybe I'm not gay; maybe I'm bisexual.) Perhaps homosexuals' ultimate fear is that somehow, at the very center of their being, they are irretrievably defective and unacceptable to society, to family, or to self. A vicious accompaniment to this fear is a kind of paranoia that people suspect or are whispering about the person's sexual orientation, which may or may not be so.

To be subjected to homophobia both from the outside via society's values and behaviors and from within via internalized hatred and fear can be devastating. At worst, it can destroy people, and it does. At best, if gay and lesbian people can process and learn from their experiences and can somehow survive, they may end up being stronger than many who have not had to contend with such oppression. Whatever the outcome, however, every gay and lesbian person develops defenses to deal with the forces and stresses of oppression.

Survival in an essentially hostile world is no small feat, and defenses are necessary to that survival. However, these same defenses often serve as primary enabling forces in the development and maintenance of alcoholism and other chemical dependencies. Thus the gay/lesbian alcoholic's defenses attain extra strength because the defenses against the disease of alcoholism and the disease of homophobia intertwine with the synergize each other. For example, alcoholics tend to isolate and distance themselves from others in order to protect their secret from being discovered. The gay or lesbian person, too, has become an artist at isolation and distancing to protect him or herself from discovery. This double dose of practice leads to a powerful defensive system.

Treating professionals therefore need to recognize and take into account certain factors. They need to acknowledge the extra power of the gay/lesbian client's defenses. They need to be mindful of distinguishing between confronting defenses that protect alcoholism and respecting defenses that serve as survival mechanisms. And they need to learn when and how to challenge a defense that seems to be obstructing treatment, even though the primary source of that defense (alcoholism, homophobia) may not be clear.

Probably the most important defense is that of denial: an essentially unconscious transforming of reality to suit the person's needs or purposes. Thus, in effect, facts as they exist in objective reality are reversed or significantly altered in the individual's subjective reality. The alcoholic's use of this extremely powerful way to defend against the painful realities of the inroads of alcoholism is well known, as is the tenacious power and effectiveness of the defense. Gays and lesbians also employ denial to combat another disease, the social disease of homophobia. They defend themselves against the onslaught of innumerable negative messages existing in objective reality. (You are sick. You are disgusting. Your sexual desires, your sexual behavior, you are unnatural. Your way of living and expressing your love is criminal.) Denial of this objective reality (and of one's self within that reality) becomes a logical, almost inevitable response. Denial becomes the shield which makes survival possible.

Living with constant negative messages about self can create enormous, often unremitting stress which is perceived and processed on both conscious and unconscious levels. Much of the stress results from the feeling of being incongruent with the surrounding world, of not belonging. Not surprisingly, many gay men and lesbians turn to and use alcohol and other drugs to assuage the pain of being incongruent or to attempt to reconcile the gulf that separates them from the majority. Thus the alcohol and drug use and addiction become an active, intrinsic part of the denial mechanism. The denial of the effects of alcoholism and/or other drug dependencies, the denial of society's homophobia, and the denial of one's homosexual identity (at least to the outside world), and sometimes the denial of one's very self these join together and synergize each other. The power of this swirling mass of denial is undeniably awesome.

Recovery from alcoholism depends in part on breaking through the denial of the disease; thus in some way confronting alcoholics' denial systems in generally standard treatment procedure. But to extrapolate from that denial experience to gay men's and lesbians' denial of homophobia is a mistake which is too often made. Gay males' and lesbians' denial of homophobia may be entirely appropriate at given times in their lives or to the treatment setting in which they find themselves. Furthermore, the removal of the anesthesia which has helped soothe their feelings of incongruency tends to expose painful nerve endings. To confront gay men or lesbians about their denial of their homosexual identity is generally irrelevant to treatment for alcoholism and can be extremely destructive, undermining treatment and sobriety. The pain generated by confronting and stripping away denial is also synergistic.

A second defensive maneuver employed by gay men and lesbians in order to maintain some sort of self-esteem is that of creating a false self which may be very different from the true self (Winnicott, 1965)[1]—that person the individual knows him/herself to be. The true self acknowledges what he or she really feels, including the capacity to feel love for and sexual response toward another member of the same sex. This true self is also painfully aware of all those harsh homophobic judgments that that capacity of love engenders in the rest of society.

[1]The following discussion is based on an adaptation of Winnicott's theories which deal with infantile and early childhood development. We have taken his concepts and applied them to later developmental issues and phases.

The false self then develops to protect the inner being by learning how to respond to homophobia, how to gather some semblance of positive reinforcement which creates the illusion of self-esteem, and how to interact with the culture's mores in a socially acceptable way. This false self can manifest itself by a person entering a heterosexual marriage and either having extramarital homosexual affairs or denying his or her sexual orientation. It can manifest itself in projecting a straight image in public and living as gay or lesbian only in private. And it can manifest itself in a constant vigilance lest anyone see the real person who lives behind the carefully developed facade.

The disparity between the true and false selves, continuing as it does over longer periods of time, often generates strong feelings of disjunction, fragmentation, confusion, and emptiness. All too often gay men and lesbians fill the void and bridge the chasm between their inner and outer selves with alcohol and/or other drugs. As the addictive process takes its course and the chemicals do their work, the person begins to experience extremely negative feelings in response to the disease process. These responses to the disease of alcoholism and to the social disease of homophobia feed, reinforce, and intensify one another. When any alcoholic stops drinking, the terrifying split between selves often haunts his/her early recovery. When gay/lesbian alcoholics stop drinking they must deal not only with problems created by the alcoholism but also with the disparity between their acceptable outer, false selves and their unacceptable (to society) inner, true selves. To push or force gay/lesbian clients to deal with this split created by homophobia or to discard the false self and disclose the true self to essential strangers is often to demand almost more than fragile alcoholic egos can bear. That many gay/lesbian alcoholics have been pushed or forced and have survived and recovered is a testament to the strength of their spirit. Many, however, did not survive.

A third defensive reaction that gay men and lesbians may have is that of hostility, anger, and rage. Again, these feelings are common also to the alcoholic condition and synergize in gay/lesbian alcoholics. For gay men and lesbians, hostility (or anger or rage) is the dragon which guards the treasure trove of the true self. Should someone come too close or try to open the door to the true self, the wrathful dragon will rise up to protect that self. Cold, unspoken rage or the kind of acid wit of *The Boys in the Band* used to try to drive off the intruder.

It is particularly important for counselors to be aware of this defense since it often emerges during treatment. What is particularly disconcerting is that hostile responses frequently are elicited by the counselor's kindness, an occurrence which counselors need to understand and reconcile for themselves. The counselor who sensitively questions the client and uncovers the client's sexual orientation may be greeted by a response such as, "Okay, now you've found me out; what're you going to do about it?" Hostile challenges conveying tremendous suspicion and mistrust need to be understood, anticipated, and meet with therapeutic equanimity.

Given that the gay/lesbian alcoholic client has defenses which may be even stronger than those of many other straight alcoholic clients, what happens to that client when he or she interacts with the treatment system? The answer is, of course, that it all depends, most particularly on the attitudes of the treatment providers. These attitudes can range from strong homophobia to empathic acceptance, and they will inform and shape the behavior of the treatment staff.

Unresolved and unchecked homophobia in staff members manifests itself in innumerable overt and covert ways. Some treatment agencies have refused to admit gay/lesbian alcoholics because of their sexual orientation. If gay/lesbian alcoholics do get past the front door, especially if their manner and behavior markedly fit the masculine female or feminine male stereotypes, the background noise during their stay on the unit may be the giggles and whispers of a frightened or repulsed staff, or they may simply be greeted with coolness or aloofness. Other forms of non-benign neglect may be that staff avoids or only half attends to the gay male or lesbian client or fails to deal with homophobic attitudes and remarks from the patient community.

Counselor's attitudes and therapy stances also may contribute to bad treatment. It can be destructive for counselors to ask such questions as, "Which role do you play?" or "Why are you gay?" It is equally destructive for counselors to make such comments as, "It makes no difference to me what you do in bed." or "We treat everybody the same here; everybody's just an alcoholic to us." Or counselors may harm their treatment relationship with the client by responding with intended kindness to the client's disclosure of gayness with a statement such as, "That doesn't matter to me." Counselors can be harmful, also, by pressuring gay or lesbian clients to reveal their sexual orientation to the group or by automatically referring clients to gay AA groups. More subtle, but no less detrimental, is to not ask clients about their sexual orientation because of the assumption that all people are heterosexual or because the counselor does not know how to deal with the answer.

The effects of such non-treatment can be illustrated by the case of Jim who, since he first tried to stop drinking at age twenty-two, has for seven years slipped in and out of sobriety, rehabilitation centers, and AA. Jim is a twenty-nine-year-old white male from a blue collar family. As the only son, a high school football hero, and the first in the family to go to college, Jim was the embodiment of his family's (especially his father's) hopes, dreams and aspirations. As he grew up, Jim always felt an uneasy awareness that the love and approval that he sought and received from his family were somehow contingent upon his fulfilling the great American dream.

Jim had his first drink at age fifteen to celebrate the end of a successful football season. He got drunk for the first time at age seventeen while on a camping trip with his best male friend when they had sex together and liked the experience. Subsequently they shared an unspoken agreement that they liked their feelings but would not discuss their behavior. In addition, they always had plenty to drink when they were together. Jim's drinking progressed but did not become a noticeable problem until he was suspended from college because of his repeated, highly visible drunkenness.

At twenty years old, rejected by his bitterly disappointed father and in need of work, Jim moved to a nearby large city, got a job in construction, and began drinking more heavily at the same time that he became more active sexually. At the age of twenty-two, Jim sought treatment for the first time, after being arrested on a DWI charge and having his boss threaten to fire him because of job performance. In the seven years since, he has been in and out of treatment and has been quite active in AA. Jim's basic pattern is to maintain sobriety for six to nine months, then relapse. Although Jim's counselors have carefully explored Jim's drinking and relapse patterns with him, he has never shared his homosexuality with them, and they have never directly asked him about his sexual orientation or even his sexual behavior. Jim has not ventured the information because he has heard the "fag jokes" on the units and has sensed the discomfort of both staff and patients in relation to sexuality in general, much less homosexuality in particular. Jim's counselors have never asked him about his sexuality because they are uncomfortable around sexual issues and because Jim is a husky, good-looking ex-footfall hero and construction worker.

After taking a geographic cure to a larger coastal city, Jim once again entered a rehabilitation center. This time was different, however, because Jim had slowly become aware of his anxiety about his homosexuality, an awareness gained by looking at his inability to have sober sex. Although desperate for guidance and support, Jim was too frightened and filled with self-hate to be able to broach the subject with anyone. Fortunately, Jim's counselor this time calmly asked many questions about Jim's significant others, his relationships, his living arrangements, and his support systems; he also took a full history, including a detailed sexual history. In the first and subsequent sessions, the counselor asked numerous questions about Jim's relapses, drinking patterns, and the meaning of his barroom activities to his life. Having established some rapport with Jim, partly by accepting Jim's evasive answers and partly by conveying his own comfort, the counselor asked Jim if he was gay and what that meant to him. At this point, good treatment had begun.

A caveat is in order here. This example is not intended to suggest that a counselor should necessarily ask directly; there are many ways to approach subjects that are difficult for clients. The point is, however, that counselors need to feel comfortable with themselves and with asking important and necessary questions so that they can attend to their clients.

Becoming a good counselor who works well with gay/lesbian alcoholics requires not only a great deal of work on attitudes and awareness levels, but also some specific skills. For instance, in numerous trainings and workshops, counselors almost invariably ask what they should say when a gay or lesbian client says to them something like, "Well, you'd drink, too, if you were gay. You don't know what it's like. You don't understand!" What helps is to ask the counselors what they would tell a client who said, "You'd drink, too, with a wife/husband/family/job, etc. like mine." Counselors who are concerned and have the best of intentions often seem to react to a gay/lesbian client as though the client were a totally unknown entity, a person so different from those within the counselors' experience that they do not know how to respond. It is helpful to become aware that while gay male and lesbian alcoholics do indeed have special issues they are, after all, just people who are alcoholics. Therefore, it is important to remember that emotional concerns and sexual issues, problems, and dysfunctions which can afflict the larger alcoholic population can and often do apply to gay/lesbian alcoholics. Gay men can become impotent as a result of their alcoholic drinking; lesbians can be pre-orgasmic; both experience decrease in sexual desire. Like straight alcoholics, they may be confused about their sexuality; terrified of intimacy; and suffer from embarrassment, shame, and guilt about sexual matters. It is helpful to keep in mind that gay male and lesbian alcoholics are more like straight alcoholics than they are like non-alcoholic gay males and lesbians.

Counselors can also benefit from examining their attitudes toward, comfort with, and knowledge about sexuality in general. Without the ability to talk with ease about sexuality, counselors will be hard pressed to be helpful to their gay/lesbian clients. In addition, counselors need to explore and decrease their own inevitable homophobic feelings, no matter how minimal those might be. It is important that they investigate their emotional reactions—are they afraid, repulsed, nervous, intolerant, angry, self-righteous, or curious? If there are any yes answers, as there are bound to be if the scrutiny is honest and thorough, then counselors can apply themselves to working through those feelings or can refer the client elsewhere. Referral is recommended if counselors feel they cannot work with a particular client.

Equally important is that counselors scrutinize their subtle, below-consciousness level stereotypes, myths, and assumptions. If a client looks like a counselor's straight friend, does that mean the client may not be gay? If a male client looks and acts very masculine, is he therefore not possibly gay? If a woman looks and acts very feminine, is she automatically not seen as possibly being a lesbian? The reverse stereotypes are much more obvious, but must still be examined. The effeminate-seeming male may not be gay; the tough, stocky woman with the short haircut may not be a lesbian. Because someone is married and has kids, could that person possibly be gay or lesbian? Other common assumptions which need to be examined are that gay men and lesbians would rather be straight if they could; that being heterosexual is better than being homosexual; that it is necessary for counselors to help their gay or lesbian clients with their sexual orientation; even when clients may not want or need help; that gay/lesbian clients always need help with their sexual orientation; that "passing" as straight is dishonest or that disclosure is necessarily good or appropriate. To investigate and challenge these stereotypes, myths and assumptions in oneself is an important task for counselors who would constructively assist their gay/lesbian clients.

In addition, it is an important learning process for counselors to meet and become acquainted with healthy gay males and lesbians to help dispel myths and stereotypes. One suggestion is to try to meet some gay/lesbian AA members and to attend some gay AA meetings. The gay social and political groups may also be a valuable source of people. Another way for counselors to enhance their effectiveness is to read materials listed on the bibliography (1983) published by the National Association of Gay Alcoholism Professionals. Learning about gay male and lesbian issues and life styles can avert the need for counselors to be taught the most rudimentary facts of gay male or lesbian life styles by their clients. Of comparable value is to learn about the coming out process by which gay men and lesbians recover from the onslaughts of homophobia and regain ownership of the self (following much the same steps as alcoholics do in recovering from alcoholism). Knowing the various stages in this process can help counselors understand where their clients may be in their life journey and what feelings they may be experiencing. Furthermore, such knowledge can enable counselors to see what the relationships may be among the clients' sexual orientation, their alcoholism, and their treatment for that alcoholism.

Other practical techniques can be helpful. Counselors can signal their acceptance by having gay/lesbian literature displayed in their offices and by obviously not tolerating homophobia in others, whether patients or staff. Counselors can learn to ask clients about sexual orientation, primarily by making questions about sexual orientation, sex partners, and significant others a routine part of the intake interview. Another method is to explain the continuum of the Kinsey scale and ask the client to place him or herself on it. Equally important is the ability to listen with a sensitive and informed ear: to what is said about significant others, residences, friends, and social activities and to what is not said (e.g., not using the pronouns "he" or "she" but instead always referring to "they").

Learning how to respond to gay/lesbian clients plays a critical role in counselors' effectiveness. Having a clear sense of how threatening disclosure may be to gay/lesbian clients helps counselors to listen with respect and heightened sensitivity when clients risk sharing their most guarded secret. At the same time, counselors need to recognize that disclosure of sexual orientation is not necessarily a prerequisite to recovery from alcoholism and indeed may have nothing to do with it. Thus counselors are well advised to challenge any belief they may hold that clients must disclose. In keeping with this is the urgent suggestion that if clients deny their homosexuality, counselors should not pursue disclosure even though they may be absolutely certain of the homosexuality. There are, of course, exceptions; but it is imperative that counselors be sure that something is an exception and that they not just automatically push when they encounter denial.

Other responses that can enhance effectiveness include tolerating clients' defensive reactions, especially their rage at the straight world for making life so miserable for them. Counselors' objectivity and support of clients in the face of these reactions can be invaluable for clients. One last caution about responding to gay/lesbian clients: counselors need to remember that they are but one link in a lifelong chain, that only a little can be done at any time. Equally important, however, is for counselors to realize that any help, support, or acceptance they may give their gay/lesbian alcoholic clients may be much more than those clients have experienced in a long time and can often help tip the balance towards sobriety.

A knowledge of and a sensitivity to some special issues is also in order. Counseling gay/lesbian alcoholics requires some awareness of the importance of discussing sober sex and the whole question of gay bars. To flatly tell gay/lesbian clients to stay out of gay bars is not always the most therapeutic move. Confidentiality is also an issue of special force because if a gay or lesbian parent's orientation becomes known, child custody is usually in jeopardy. Other special issues include how and when to advise going to gay or mainstream AA meetings; how to assist clients in finding good sponsors (e.g., sometimes a gay male will ask a straight woman to sponsor him); how to help clients deal with the issue of honesty in AA in relation to the fear (and possible fact) of rejection; and how to advise clients who may be suffering from a strong dose of religious guilt. Obviously it is critically important for counselors to know what resources are available and to have good contacts in the AA community.

Two final comments may be made about providing treatment to gay male and lesbian alcoholics. If counselors are afraid to or do not want to work with gay/lesbian clients, then they should not do so. No treatment is better than inept or hostile treatment. If, however, counselors are willing to examine and work on their attitudes and make whatever changes are necessary, then they can have the satisfaction of knowing that their caring and concern can play a special and critically important part in gay/lesbian alcoholics' recoveries.

REFERENCES

American Psychiatric Association. *Diagnostic and Statistical Manual of Mental Disorders* (3rd ed.). Washington, D.C.: Author, 1980.

Bieber, I., Dain, H., Dince, P., Drellich, M., Grand H., Gundlach, R., Kremer, M., Rifkin, A., Wilbur, C., & Bieber, T. *Homosexuality: A Psychoanalytic Study.* New York: Basic Books, 1962.

Kinsey, A., Pomeroy, W., Martin, C. *Sexual Behavior of the Human Male.* Philadelphia: W.B. Saunders Co., 1948.

Kinsey, A., Pomeroy, W., Martin C., & Gebhart, P. *Sexual Behavior in the Human Female.* Philadelphia: W.B. Saunders Co., 1953.

Knutson, D. Introduction. In D. Knutson (Ed.,) *Homosexuality and the Law* (Vol. 1 of the Monograph Series, *Research on Homosexuality*). New York: The Haworth Press, 1980.

Myers, M. Counseling the Parents of Young Homosexual Male Patients. *Journal of Homosexuality*, 1981/82, 7 (2/3), 131–141.

National Association of Gay Alcoholism Professionals. *NAGAP Bibliography*: Resources on Alcoholism and *Lesbians/Gay Men* (Rev. Ed.). New York: Author, 1983.

Vetri, D. The Legal Arena: Progress for Gay Civil Rights. In D. Knutson (Ed.), *Homosexuality and the Law* (Vol. 1 of the Monograph Series, *Research on Homosexuality*). New York: The Haworth Press, 1980.

Weinberg, G. *Society and the Healthy Homosexual.* Garden City, N.Y.: Anchor Press/Doubleday, 1972.

Winnicott, D. Ego Distortion in Terms of True and False Self. In D. Winnicott, *The Maturational Process and the Facilitating Environment.* New York: International Universities Press, Inc., 1965.

Sexual Dynamics
of the Client-Counselor Relationship

Jerry Edelwich, M.S.W.
Archie Brodsky, B.A.

A subject that receives insufficient attention in training programs for alcoholism counselors, as in other human service professions (Edelwich & Brodsky, 1982), is the sexual dynamics that complicate the relationship between counselor and client. In psychoanalytic terms, sexual feelings that arise in the course of counseling can be seen as expressions of transference (whereby the client reacts to the counselor as a surrogate for "significant others" in the client's life) and countertransference (whereby the counselor reacts to the client on the basis of similar associations). Alternately, these feelings can be understood as manifestations of the sexual energy that can arise between any two people, here intensified by the intimacy of the therapeutic exchange and by the special vulnerability that exists for the client and sometimes for the counselor as well. Whatever their origins, these potentially disruptive emotional currents are ever present in the working life of an alcoholism counselor. If not dealt with appropriately, they can lead to less effective client care; breaches of ethics; and emotional, professional, and/or legal problems for the counselor. Yet most counselors learn to cope with these dynamics only through difficult on-the-job experience.

In order to increase awareness and facilitate better training in this sensitive area, we will explore how the cross-currents of sexuality manifest themselves in counseling situations, what personal and clinical dilemmas they produce, and what can be done about them when they arise. The overtures, reactions, denials, hidden agendas, and limit-testing that simmer beneath the surface of a counseling session can be summarized under five overlapping themes: (1) seduction; (2) power; (3) opportunity; (4) self-interest; (5) morality. Under the last of these headings we will propose ethical guidelines to be applied by counselors, trainees, teachers, trainers, and supervisors.

SEDUCTION

There are as many different kinds of seduction as there are ways of projecting one's sexuality (overtly or covertly) to attain a desired end. It is the nature of human interaction that people are drawn into emotional involvements which support or interfere with the avowed purposes of the individuals concerned. In this broad sense, seduction is not inherently bad and need not be focused on concrete sexual aims. Scheflen (1965) analyzes therapy itself as a "quasi-courtship" in which the feelings that arise between the counselor and client create an atmosphere favorable to constructive change on the client's part. In psychoanalysis the patient is 'seduced' into a transference relationship, again in the service of self-knowledge and personal growth. However, the seduction we are concerned with here, whether or not it is acted out through sexual contact, involves sexual attractions and gestures that work against the purposes of counseling.

A textbook case of seduction in this sense is the following (adapted from Edelwich & Brodsky, 1982):

A 30-year-old woman is referred to employee assistance for possible alcohol abuse after a period of declining job performance. She is referred to a male counselor in his twenties with six months' experience. During her first several sessions the woman does not admit alcohol or other drug use, but does complain of numerous personal problems (which are also the subject of frequent after-hours calls to a crisis line). In the weeks that follow she becomes less withdrawn, but when confronted with difficult questions she responds with tears, confused utterances, or flirtatious behavior. She flirts by moving her eyes so as to establish eye contact with the counselor while rearranging herself to expose more of her body. The counselor, assuming this behavior to be deliberate, confronts her about it. She denies conscious intent, stating instead that "it just happens" when she feels defensive. She observes that people tend to lose track of the conversation when their attention is drawn from her face to another part of her body.

The counselor, concerned to maintain his therapeutic stance, consults with his supervisor, who warns him to be prepared for an escalation from physical to verbal overtures. At her next session the client says, "You know, you've helped me a lot in a short time. You seem so confident; your life seems so squared away; you don't have problems like I do." She then tells the counselor that she finds him attractive and desires a sexual relationship with him.

His discomfort evident, the inexperienced counselor replies that the professional relationship does not allow for intimate personal contact. The issue is not discussed further, but the counselor continues to have disturbing thoughts. "She's God's gift to counselors," he says to himself. "If ever I wanted an affair 'on the side,' here's my opportunity." He realizes, however, that if he acted on this fantasy, he might be destroying his career and his marriage. He goes back to his supervisor, who questions him about his reaction to the client's flattery. "I have to admit," the counselor says, "that it was a big blowup for my ego."

The supervisor reviews with the counselor whether the client has made sufficient progress to justify continuing the sessions. They decide to establish stricter guidelines, including a specified agenda for each session and the elimination of after-hours calls.

This case illustrates several typical features of client-counselor sexual dynamics, some of which run counter to sensationalistic stereotypes. The client's behavior issues not from a calculated strategy but from an unconscious pattern of avoidance of difficult personal issues (especially her drinking and its consequences). For his part, the counselor is not an unethical exploiter of unwary patients, but rather a well-intentioned person whose inexperience prevents him from proceeding confidently when his self-esteem and self-interest are engaged. He is susceptible to flattery even while he recognizes that sexual acting out with a client not only is unethical, but also represents a threat to both his personal and professional life. Although he does not act improperly, he is unsure of himself. In his preoccupation with his own discomfort he misses the opportunity to explore the client's behavior therapeutically (as by saying, "Let's talk about this—why do you want to have a love affair with me?"). He minimizes the damage, however, by consulting with his supervisor; twice the case shows the value of supervisory intervention.

How Clients Seduce

Quick recognition of seductive behavior makes it easier for the counselor to respond effectively. The following types of seductive behavior and signs of seductive intent are familiar to experienced counselors:

Fantasy. Fantasy is the first step toward sexual involvement. In itself, however, it is harmless, private, and invisible. Only when it begins to be acted upon does it become a problem, and then it is no longer fantasy.

Preference for counselors of a particular gender. Clients who are predisposed to confuse professional with personal relationships tend to choose counselors of the sex to which they are attracted. Administrators of treatment facilities can expect to see clients express this bias by circumventing assignment to counselors of the ''wrong'' gender.

Edited self-presentation. Clients sometimes seek to present a favorable image of themselves to counselors of the sex to which they are attracted. This personal agenda interferes with the full disclosure required in the counseling situation.

Voyeurism. Inappropriate interest in the counselor's personal life should be regarded as a danger signal. "Are you married?" or "Do you have a lover?" is often merely the first in a chain of inquiries that culminates in a sexual offer.

Extracurricular contacts. Unscheduled office visits and frequent phone calls serve as a warning to the counselor that a client's interest may be more than professional.

Verbal exhibitionism. When clients recount their sexual exploits at length and in graphic physical detail, they may simply be trying to distract the counselor's attention from serious therapeutic exploration. (Homosexual practices in particular can have great shock value for the uninitiated.) However, they may also be making (implicitly or explicitly) a sexual pitch to the counselor, one that says, in effect, "Wouldn't you like to be the person I do these things with?"

Body language. An attempt at seduction usually begins with physical cues, which may progress from the visual to the tactile. These include revealing dress (tight or open garments), suggestive poses, eye contact, touching one's own body (e.g., stroking one's legs), and physical contact with the counselor (e.g., bumping knees, touching hands).

Spoken invitations. Compliments directed at the counselor's attractiveness, skill, or enviable position in life often lead to a sexual invitation. The client may also probe for the counselor's personal dissatisfactions. A counselor who answers the question "Are you happily married?" (even in the affirmative) opens the door for the client to reply, "How happy? I can make you happier."

The styles of client seduction reflect the sex role stereotypes of the larger society: the passive style, in which the client projects "learned helplessness" (Seligman, 1975); and the active or "macho" style, in which the client seeks to overwhelm (and perhaps intimidate) the counselor. The traditional association of these roles with the female and male genders respectively is still observable, although it is breaking down.

Why Clients Seduce

Clients have so many reasons to act seductively toward counselors that it can be difficult to attribute such behavior in a given instance to one motivation as distinct from several others (Shochet et al., 1976). The following motivations, which should be understood to be overlapping, are those most frequently cited by counselors:

To express sexual attraction or gratify sexual desire. Sometimes there is nothing more to a client's sexual interest in a counselor than the effect of proximity to an attractive person. People who happen to be clients occasionally are attracted to people who happen to be counselors (and vice versa). But clients often act seductively toward counselors at whom they would not look twice on the street. Seduction is such a pervasive pattern of client behavior, even when the counselor's age or appearance makes the attraction implausible, that explanations must be sought elsewhere. In the words of Hollender and Shevitz (1978, p. 776), "The main issue is not the nature of the patient's provocativeness but what is being sought: almost never a sexual relationship and almost always special attention or nurturance."

To divert attention from treatment issues. Perhaps the most important function of seductive words and gestures is to divert one's own and/or the counselor's attention from anxiety-provoking therapeutic issues. Although this pattern of evasion can occur in any kind of therapy, it is especially common in alcoholism counseling, where it fits in with the alcoholic's denial and manipulativeness. Sometimes the sexual diversion is a largely unconscious by-product of the client's anxiety. In one such case, as reported by the counselor, a 19-year-old woman who denied her alcohol problem "went through the usual defenses—tears, avoidance, anger. She tried to walk out twice. Then she started working the sexual angle." In other cases the client has the conscious purpose of distracting the counselor from the issues at hand, as when a male client confronted on his drinking by a female counselor repeatedly interrupted with remarks such as "You have really nice eyes" and "You have such a calming effect on me."

To bribe or manipulate. The attempt by a client to use sex as a quid pro quo for favored treatment is found less in open-ended, exploratory therapies than in therapies directed toward a specific form of compliance, such as alcoholism counseling. Sex is either the price to be paid for the client's compliance ("I won't drink if you'll play ball with me") or, more commonly, the counselor's payoff for not exacting compliance ("I'll play ball with you if you'll let me get away with a drink now and then"). Typically, the bargain is not struck in such straightforward terms. Instead, the client may seek leniency in return for flattery and the pleasantries of flirtation, the implicit message being, "If you don't give me a hard time, I'll go on being as sweet and agreeable as I am now." Alternately, in the "maybe someday" approach, sex is dangled before the counselor as a possible future reward. Here the client is saying, in effect, "If you'll look the other way, if you'll tell me what I want to hear (that I'll be able to drink safely again), maybe you and I can get it together some time."

To seek favoritism in conjoint therapy. In marital, family, or couple counseling, one partner will often use seductive techniques to gain the counselor's allegiance against the spouse or other participants.

To compromise the counselor's position. Although a client can suffer great emotional damage from sexual involvement with a counselor, a manipulative client may take (or ignore) that risk to gain an advantage in a perceived power struggle with the counselor. A counselor who has been seduced is one who can be blackmailed. It is difficult to confront (especially in a group) a client who is also a lover.

To gain status among one's peers. Clients in residential treatment facilities may seek to maintain an image among other residents by boasting about the real or imaginary affairs with counselors. Although here the intention is not to compromise the counselor professionally, that may, unfortunately, be the result.

To partake of the counselor's perceived strength. The alcoholic client, while perhaps living a highly developed life in certain areas, in other respects has not progressed very far along the hierarchies of needs identified by Maslow (1954) and Glasser (1976). A person who is dealing with basic survival issues (whether emotional, financial, or both) is susceptible to magical thoughts such as "I might be okay if only this strong, successful person were taking care of me all the time instead of just an hour a week." From the client's vantage point the counselor appears as powerful, autonomous, accomplished, and self-assured. Sexual bonding seems a natural way for the client to take on these qualities. This parentification of the counselor is akin to the "transference neurosis" in psychoanalysis, whereby the association of the analyst with the patient's prior love objects causes the patient to focus obsessively on the analyst as a person.

To gain attention and gratification through the use of accustomed strategies. Finally, clients are seductive simply because they are clients. A client's behavior in counseling reveals inadequate coping strategies learned earlier in life. The learned helplessness, the manipulation of dependency, the deviousness, the corrupt bargains, the diversion of attention, the sexist caricatures—these are the deviant skills that have brought the alcoholic to the point of needing help in the first place. The counselor's response, therefore, should be therapeutic rather than judgmental.

How Counselors Unwittingly Contribute to Seduction

For the client, the counseling relationship is highly charged emotionally. Clients see and feel deep meanings even when none are intended. It is all the more important, then, for the counselor to avoid ambiguous communications or unwittingly provocative actions. Counselors who have no sexual designs on clients may be 'seduced into seducing' by their own impulses together with a client's behavior. Insufficient training and experience can be a factor as well. The following are some ways in which counselors are embroiled in the game of seduction:

Attraction to clients. It is normal for a counselor to feel an attraction to a client. However, it is unethical to act on the attraction, and it is unprofessional to allow oneself to be distracted from the job of counseling by such feelings.

Wishful thinking and self-seduction. An inexperienced counselor typically will come to a supervisor with a detailed rundown of a client's dress, complexion, eye color, and so forth, and then remark, "It was difficult to keep my mind on therapy." However normal the feeling of attraction, the counselor whose mind wanders in this way is not giving the client the professional attention to which the client (even one who provokes the distraction) is entitled. Counselors who lack formal training are more likely to dwell on their clients' appearance and behavior than are those with a professional background. One who indulges such musings may go on to tease oneself with impossible dreams and to rationalize behavior that puts both oneself and the client in a vulnerable position (e.g., sitting too close during a session, meeting the client after hours).

Ambiguous communications. Counselors express warmth and caring in both verbal and nonverbal ways. The counselor who is insufficiently alert to the nuances of both kinds of communication may convey mixed messages, whether by sitting with knees touching the client's or by appearing to leave open the possibility of sexual rewards for therapeutic progress ("Well, not now, but maybe somewhere down the road, if you stop drinking . . . . "). Clarity of expression is essential. "You are an attractive person" is an acceptable professional communication; "I'm attracted to you" is not.

Voyeurism. Counselors who are plagued with clients' elaborate recitals of their sexual activities may learn, through supervision or their own therapy, that they are unconsciously encouraging such exhibitionism. Clients can sense the difference between appropriate therapeutic inquiries and inappropriate personal ones, such as "What did you do next? Did you enjoy it? Are there any things you won't do?" Some clients are distressed by this voyeurism and may leave counseling because of it. Others 'play to the gallery,' taking advantage of the counselor's complicity in their own agenda of extratherapeutic diversion.

Overidentification. Counselors are at risk for establishing too close (or too distant) a relationship with a client who presents issues similar to those that remain unresolved in the counselor's own life. A counselor who, through inexperience, youthful idealism, or emotional vulnerability, identifies too closely with a client's feelings may be unwilling to confront a seductive client.

Power has a dual function in relation to sex. Power is used to gain sexual rewards, and sex is used as a token in the struggle for power. These elemental dynamics play themselves out in counseling as well as other life situations.

The Client's Power Versus the Counselor's

The client and counselor bring different (and usually unequal) kinds of power to the therapeutic interchange. The client's power is personal and physical. It is the power to attract with charm and dynamism or to intimidate with the threat of violence, sexual or otherwise. Many alcoholic clients have a record of violent behavior that makes this threat credible. Violence-prone male clients often are more threatened by male than by female counselors, and some may feel inhibited from striking a woman. Even then, however, the client may seek to establish ascendancy over the counselor with sexual machismo (e.g., touching or grabbing.) These gestures should be understood as an assertion of what little power is at hand in a situation of relative powerlessness.

To the extent that the client perceives a counseling session to be a power struggle, the power arrayed against the client is not only personal, but social and institutional as well. The counselor is a certified representative of institutions that impact directly on the client's life. The counselor not only has access to the client's file, but adds entries to the file that may affect whether the client is discharged from a hospital or residential treatment center, obtains or keeps a job, stays in military service, goes to prison, or receives disability payments. Power in this sense lies in the possession and transmission of privileged information. Another type of power, as discussed above, resides in the counselor's very being; that of a strong, successful person who "has the answers." All told, the counselor has considerable leverage that can be used or abused.

Legitimate and Illegitimate Uses of Power

A young female counselor in an alcoholism treatment center found that she was getting good results by responding graciously to her male clients' "gentlemanly" gestures and overtures. The positive tone of her relationships with clients improved morale and appeared to contribute to her client's progress. Still, she told her supervisor that she had misgivings about this "manipulation" of clients. Her supervisor told her that therapeutic seductiveness was a

legitimate tool in a counselor's repertoire—provided that it was
used solely in the client's interest, that the stated purposes of counseling were served, and that there was not the slightest hint of present or future availability for a sexual or otherwise inappropriate personal relationship.

The distinction between legitimate and illegitimate use of the
counselor's power to "seduce" has been summarized as follows:
"To seduce a client into experiencing the natural consequences of
responsible behavior by interposing the immediate reward of pleas-
ing the [counselor] is acceptable therapeutic technique. To indulge a
client in the wish that good behavior will earn a sexual reward is to
compromise the [counselor's] power and ultimately disillusion the
client" (Edelwich & Brodsky, 1982, p. 46).

OPPORTUNITY

Sexual opportunity in counseling situations arises out of human
vulnerability, and it works both sides of the street. The client's vulnerability is the counselor's opportunity, and the counselor's vulnerability is the client's opportunity. Typically, the exploitation of
opportunities is neither systematic nor one-sided. Rather, the client
and counselor half-consciously exploit each other's vulnerability
while acting out their own (Chodoff, 1968).

Client's Vulnerability—Counselor's Opportunity

The vulnerability of the client stems from disadvantages in life
that have led to inadequate or dysfunctional learning. People who
have not learned to make constructive choices for themselves are
susceptible to the appeal of shortcuts to gratification and fulfillment
such as substance abuse and crime. Other such shortcuts are to yield
to an abuse of the counselor's power or to attempt to use sex to "get
to" a counselor.

A graphic example of the vulnerability the client exhibits and of
how it translates into opportunity for the counselor is provided by a
homosexual male counselor who works with fellow homosexual alcoholics:

> I am in a position to play around with my clients (if I wanted
> to) for the same reasons that I once was putty in the hands of

my own therapist. I'm their kind of person in two ways, and on top of that I have the serenity that they're seeking. They depend on me to tell them how I got sober, especially in gay circumstances. (Edelwich and Brodsky, 1982, p. 52)

The client has found certain doors closed in life, and the counselor appears to hold the keys. Therein lies the opportunity to hold improper personal sway as well as exert positive moral persuasion.

The temptation to take advantage of client's vulnerability is especially strong in residential treatment communities, prisons, and any other environment where the counseling staff has continuous (rather than scheduled) access to residents or inmates. Here, where the institution serves as a total environment for residents, the combination of (typically) adolescent or young adult residents, counselors without much formal clinical training, and strong peer pressures on both residents and counselors creates an explosive situation. Abuses have been reported in such settings both with male counselors and female clients and vice versa. These abuses do not necessarily involve actual sexual contact. In one case female residents left the female counselors to whom they were assigned and flocked to male counselors with whom they spent unscheduled hours responding to voyeuristic questions with titillating confessions. In scenarios such as this the vulnerability and the exploitation are mutual. Consequently, the need for vigilant monitoring and supervision is especially great.

Counselor's Vulnerability—Client's Opportunity

Counselors, too, are vulnerable human beings. They have their good days and bad days, their life crises and discontents. People enter the counseling field carrying what one experienced clinician has described as "an empty cup." The empty cup stands for a range of needs—for accomplishments, recognition, control, self-knowledge, love—that must be satisfied before the counselor can effectively serve others. The cup is filled as the counselor matures on the job, but even then there are setbacks, disillusionments, and incomplete satisfactions.

Any of a number of unfulfilled needs, personal and professional, can make a counselor vulnerable to inappropriate intimacies with clients (Chodoff, 1968; Dahlberg, 1970; Marmor, 1976). Marital problems, divorce, breakup with a lover, anything that makes for a lack of intimate fulfillment is an obvious instance. One who seeks a dependent partner to satisfy one's own need for intimacy (Peele & Brodsky, 1976) may find such a partner in an emotionally vulnerable client. The various frustrations that contribute to job burnout (Edelwich & Brodsky, 1980) can also motivate a counselor to seek compensatory gratifications. Among these are career stagnation, frustration at a lack of visible accomplishment, case overload, client recidivism, bureaucratic obstacles, and inadequate funding. Whatever isolates the counselor from normal social and professional contacts—long hours, six- and seven-day work weeks, geographical remoteness, private practice, live-in responsibilities at a residential center—may exacerbate emotional needs and undermine ethical judgment. These vulnerabilities can lead the counselor to react carelessly to the gifts, dinner invitations, and phone calls at home by which clients test the counselor's limits. That carelessness in turn opens the way to opportunity for the client.

Insufficient training and experience constitute another major factor in the counselor's vulnerability. In the alcoholism treatment field, the risks are highest for paraprofessional counselors whose primary qualifications are enthusiasm and a personal history of alcoholism. A male counselor who has been sober for just six months, who is underpaid and overworked, who sees his clients relapse and his recommendations ignored by professional staff, who has unresolved issues concerning women, and who might not be otherwise employable may well seek relief from the stresses of the job by exploiting his female clients. Currently, the potential for abuses of this kind is being reduced by the professionalization of alcoholism counseling. Although personal experience with alcoholism can be an enormous asset for the counselor, it is most effectively applied in conjunction with (rather than instead of) professional skills and certification. The professionally qualified counselor is still subject to wayward impulses but is less able to rationalize (or expect to get away with) acting on them than is the paraprofessional (Silverstein et al., 1981).

SELF-INTEREST

Opportunity is always there, but to act in one's own interest is a choice. Ideally, clients would see it as in their best interest to attend to the business of treatment, but if clients always interpreted their self-interest appropriately they would not need counselors. Thus, a client may opt to manipulate the situation, whether for sexual gratification, temporary emotional fulfillment, dispensation from the requirements of treatment, or an "edge" in the counseling relationship. A counselor, too, can choose to seize upon opportunity for immediate personal gain. Unlike the client, however, the counselor must attempt to rationalize this clear violation of professional ethics.

Rationalizing Self-Interest

Some counselors, like other helping professionals, come up with ingenious rationalizations for acting out sexually with clients. They claim that it is an expression of warmth and caring, a mark of personal respect, a courtesy to spare the client the pain of rejection, or a form of therapeutic involvement (applied selectively to young, attractive clients of one gender). In the view of all reputable commentators, these rationalizations are invalidated by the very nature of therapy or counseling. A therapeutic relationship rests on complete trust. The counselor, like a nurturing parent, provides a safe space in which the client can be fully revealing (of, among other things, weakness, dependency, and irrationality) without fear that this openness will be exploited. The mutual revelation, intimacy, and added vulnerability of a sexual relationship plainly violate this special space of caring "neutrality" (Dahlberg, 1970; Kardener, 1974; Marmor, 1972; Silverstein, 1977).

This point need hardly be belabored. There are, however, subtler forms of self-interest engaged in by decent people who have no wish to act unethically and no awareness that they may be doing so. For example, a male counselor who has never had sexual relations with a client in treatment gives the following account of his dealings with former clients:

> I've gone out with a couple of former clients when they had been sober for over a year and had been away from my agency for an equivalent period of time. I had introduced them to A.A., and by that point I thought of them as A.A. friends rather than clients. They were well into their recovery; it was almost as if they had become different people. (Edelwich & Brodsky, 1982, p. 94)

However plausible his reasoning and however harmless his actions, this well-intentioned counselor is rationalizing self-interest. He takes his clients to A.A., terminates them (though not prematurely) as clients, sees them at A.A. meetings, and declares them to be friends. This man may well be conscientious enough not to allow his treatment of clients to be affected by the possibility of seeing them socially later. Given that option, however, a less scrupulous counselor might deliberately take on and then terminate clients as a way of recruiting sexual partners.

Agencies employing counselors generally do not place restrictions on sexual involvements with ex-clients after an appropriate interval (whatever that may be) has elapsed. Nonetheless, there are strong grounds for discouraging such conduct as a matter of policy, to be questioned only in extraordinary cases. Three major considerations make intimacies with former clients inadvisable.

1. *Compromise of the treatment process.* A counselor who allows for the possibility of a love affair after termination may have difficulty maintaining clinical objectivity during the course of treatment. With later personal rewards in view, the counselor may "pull punches" by avoiding difficult issues. Every aspect of treatment from initiation to termination can be compromised by undisciplined countertransference feelings.

2. *Denial of future therapeutic support.* Once the therapeutic relationship is exchanged for a personal one, the ex-client can never come back to the same counselor for further treatment if needed. Although one can turn to other counselors, the secure trust and permanent availability—the island of safety—offered by the original therapeutic relationship are irrevocably lost.

3. *Undermining of the personal relationship.* A healthy intimate involvement is a relationship between equals. A counselor-client relationship with privileged information passing in one direction only is not. This inequality can be extremely difficult to overcome. It remains as a memory that can be revived at moments of stress, as when the counselor-turned-lover exclaims, "I knew you back when you were drinking!"

There may be some very rare instances in which these arguments are outweighed by the potential for a loving union between two people who happen to be a counselor and former client. To avoid the pitfalls of rationalization, a supervisor should be involved in the determination of whether a particular case is an exceptional relationship.

Countervailing Self-Interest: What the Counselor Stands to Lose

The relative infrequency of outright sexual abuse of clients by helping professionals (Holroyd & Brodsky, 1977; Kardener et al.,

1973) is attributable not only to personal and professional ethics, but to the conflicting imperatives of the counselor's self-interest. Although one's immediate self-interest may lie in an improper liaison, one's long-term interest argues for restraint. Considerations that would give most counselors pause include limitations of time and energy, awareness that romantic infatuation is time-limited, and the threat to one's marriage and family life. Also placed in jeopardy are one's job and perhaps career. The higher one's professional standing and income (and the more time and effort it took to achieve it), the more one has to lose. This is another reason why professional training and certification of alcoholism counselors stand to reduce the incidence of unethical conduct in this field. Finally, there is an increasing risk of legal liability for abuse of the counseling relationship (Gutheil & Appelbaum, 1982; Halleck, 1980; Mason & Stitham, 1977; Stone, 1976).

MORALITY

Ideas about what is good and right can affect counseling and its sexual undercurrents in different ways. They can stand between the client and counselor as an obstacle to good treatment, or they can point the way to a clear resolution of the sexual dilemmas of counseling.

Moralistic Reactions

Counselors and clients have their personal moral standards just as anyone else does. When these clash, however, treatment can suffer. As a case in point, a young male homosexual came to a middle-aged female counselor for treatment for alcoholism. The counselor was so intent on treating the client's homosexuality (for which he did not seek treatment) that she practically ignored his alcoholism. This counselor imposed her own moral agenda on the client. It would have been more professional for her to limit her intervention to the avowed agenda of the client and the agency.

Similarly, moralistic reactions to seductive behavior directed toward the counselor can also be detrimental to therapy. It is understandable that the counselor may be personally offended by such behavior but, to act on one's revulsion or outrage is as unprofessional as to act on an attraction to a client. Seduction, like other desperate strategies, is to be expected from a client, and the appropriate response to it is therapeutic, not punitive.

Ethical Guidelines

Although the counselor's personal morality may be a mixed blessing for the client and for treatment, another kind of morality—i.e., professional ethics—is an indispensable guide. As discussed above, the ethics of the counseling profession dictate an absolute prohibition of sexual relations with clients currently in treatment and extreme caution concerning intimacies with former clients. Where most counselors have problems, however, is not with these actual transgressions. Rather, it is in the gray area of day-to-day temptations, uncertainties, and upsets that counselors seek ethical and clinical guidance. How does one respond to "leading questions," "come-ons," and other provocative behavior on the part of a client? How does one keep one's own feelings of attraction under control so as to keep one's mind on counseling?

The "dos and don'ts" listed here represent a distillation of the experience of counselors and other helping professionals in negotiating the troubled waters of client-counselor relations. (For further discussion of each guideline see Edelwich & Brodsky, 1982.) The list is followed by a brief summary of a few basic guidelines and the principles underlying them.

- DO acknowledge your own feelings.
- DO separate your personal feelings from dealings with the client.
- DO confide in your supervisors, peers, or therapist.
- DO set limits while giving the client a safe space for self-expression.
- DO express non-sexual caring.
- DO confront the issue straightforwardly.
- DO explore the client's behavior therapeutically.
- DON'T make the client's problems your own.
- DON'T give your problems to the client.
- DON'T be rejecting.
- DON'T be drawn into answering personal questions or giving the client other "double messages."

It comes as a relief to many counselors that personal reactions to clients, including sexual attraction, need not be repressed, denied, or explained away. Being a counselor does not exempt one from normal human feelings. If psychoanalysts have sexual fantasies about clients, so can alcoholism counselors. Simply acknowledging one's feelings can greatly reduce the strain of (and resistance to) coping with them.

Having acknowledged one's feelings, whether one acts or does not act on them is a choice; to refrain from acting them out unprofessionally is a responsibility. While clients may need to learn that they have the capacity to make choices, the counselor is assumed to be able to exercise that capacity—i.e., to accept the responsibility of acting in the client's interest regardless of any distractions or disturbances, attractions or aversions, that may occur along the way (Ellis & Harper, 1975; Glasser, 1965; Simon, Howe, & Kirschenbaum, 1972). Anyone who is paid to treat clients takes on this obligation; professional training and credentials simply strengthen one's hand in doing so. Initially, the assumption sounds forbidding that one has, without qualification, the power to choose. In fact, it is liberating and empowering. Once grasped, it enables one to set aside with a minimum of energy and emotional investment those attractions that are not appropriately acted on, so that one remains both human and professional (Dahlberg, 1970; Winnicott, 1960).

The counselor should avoid not only compromising situations with a client (e.g., dinners out, meetings away from the office or clinic), but also compromising lines of conversation initiated by a client's limit-testing. To answer questions about one's personal life is to step into a trap where each answer invites further intrusion, as in this exchange:

Client: "Do you have a lover?"

Counselor: "No, not at this time."

Client: "Do you miss it?"

One need not and should not make excuses for turning down a date with a client. Don't say, "I'm too busy" (another time you might not be). Don't say, "I have a steady relationship with someone" (you might not always have one). Don't say (to a homosexual client), "Sorry, but I'm heterosexual" (would you tell a heterosexual client that you're homosexual?). The counselor does not need to play the client's seductive games. Rather, a therapeutic focus on the client's feelings and motives should be maintained.

A counselor who is troubled by strong, persistent feelings of attraction to a client should not burden the client, who already has enough problems, with this personal issue. Instead, the counselor should consult with a supervisor, with peers or colleagues, or with the counselor's own therapist or counselor. In difficult cases a supervisor may hold conjoint sessions to work out the problem with the client and counselor together.

A wise supervisor also will discourage the panacea of referring difficult clients (including those to whom the client feels sexually attracted) to another counselor or agency. Except in extreme instances where the client would be harmed by continued involvement with the same counselor, referral amounts to a kind of buck-passing, for somebody eventually will have to take care of the client. Routine referrals represent a denial both of the counselor's capacity to make free choices and of the counselor's responsibility to the client. The counselor who evades clinical and ethical challenges by referring them out misses the opportunity to grow professionally, to provide ongoing professional support for the client, and to engage the client in a therapeutic exploration of the behavior in question. Thus the cynical slogan, "When in doubt, refer out," might better be rephrased, "Don't refer out—work it out."

REFERENCES

Chodoff, P. The seductive patient. *Medical Aspects of Human Sexuality*, 1968, *2*(2), 52–55.

Dahlberg, C.C. Sexual contact between patient and therapist. Contemporary Psychoanalysis, 1970, *6*, 107–124.

Edelwich, J., & Brodsky, A. *Burnout: Stages of Disillusionment in the Helping Professions.* New York: Human Sciences Press, 1980.

Edelwich, J., & Brodsky, A. *Sexual Dilemmas for the Helping Professional.* New York: Brunner/Mazel, 1982.

Ellis, A., & Harper, R.A. *A New Guide to Rational Living.* N. Hollywood, Cal.: Wilshire, 1975.

Glasser, W. *Reality Therapy.* New York: Harper & Row, 1965.

Glasser, W. *Positive Addiction.* New York: Harper & Row, 1976.

Gutheil, T.G., & Appelbaum, P.S. *Clinical Handbook of Psychiatry and the Law.* New York: McGraw-Hill, 1982.

Halleck, S.L. *Law in the Practice of Psychiatry: A Handbook for Clinicians.* New York: Plenum, 1980.

Hollender, M.H., & Shevitz, S. The seductive patient. *Southern Medical Journal*, 1978, *71*, 776–778.

Holroyd, J.C., & Brodsky, A.M. Psychologists' attitudes and practices regarding erotic and nonerotic physical contact with patients. *American Psychologist*, 1977, *32*, 843–849.

Kardener, S.H. Sex and the physician-patient relationship. *American Journal of Psychiatry*, 1974, *131*, 1134–1136.

Kardener, S.H., Fuller, M., & Mensh, I.N. A survey of physicians' attitudes and practices regarding erotic and nonerotic contact with patients. *American Journal of Psychiatry*, 1973, *130*, 1077–1081.

Marmor, J. Sexual acting-out in psychotherapy. *American Journal of Psychoanalysis*, 1972, *32*, 3–8.

Marmor, J. Some psychodynamic aspects of the seduction of patients in psychotherapy. *American Journal of Psychoanalysis*, 1976, *36*, 319–323.

Maslow, A.H. *Motivation and Personality.* New York: Harper, 1954.

Mason, P.E., & Stitham, M.D. The expensive dalliance: assessing the cost of patient-therapist sex. *Bulletin of the American Academy of Psychiatry and the Law,* 1977, *5,* 450–455.

Peele, S., & Brodsky, A. *Love and Addiction.* New York: New American Library, 1976.

Scheflen, A.E. Quasi-courtship behavior in psychotherapy. *Psychiatry,* 1965, *28,* 245–257.

Seligman, M.E.P. *Helplessness: On Depression, Development, and Death.* San Francisco: W.H. Freeman, 1975.

Shochet, B.R., Levin, L., Lowen, M., & Lisansky, E.T. Roundtable: dealing with the seductive patient. *Medical Aspects of Human Sexuality,* 1976, *10*(12), 90–104.

Silverstein, L.M. *Consider the Alternative.* Minneapolis: CompCare Publications, 1977.

Silverstein, L.M., Edelwich, J., Flanagan, D., & Brodsky, A. *High on Life: A Story of Addiction and Recovery.* Hollywood, Fla.: Health Communications, 1981.

Simon, S.B., Howe, L.W., & Kirschenbaum, H. *Values Clarification.* New York: Hart, 1972.

Stone, A.A. *Mental Health and Law: A System in Transition.* New York: Jason Aronson, 1976.

Winnicott, D.W. Countertransference. *British Journal of Medical Psychology,* 1960, *33,* 17–21.

Glossary*

Technical Term	Street Term	Meaning/Function
Amenorrhea		A lack of menstruation.
Anal intercourse	Corn husking	Placing the penis into the anus of a man or a woman.
Androgen		Male hormone, i.e., testosterone, produced in the testes.
Asexual		Behavior which avoids overt sexual contact.
Bisexual	AD/DC	Anatomically: having sexual organs of both sexes. Behaviorally: having sexual interest in both sexes.
Castration		Removal of the testes in men or the ovaries in women.
Celibacy		Abstaining from sexual activity.
Cervix		Part of the uterus.
Circumcision		Surgical removal of the penis foreskin.

*Adapted from Hartman, Quinn, Young, 1981.

Climax	Shoot your wad, to come	An orgasm.
Clitoris	Clit	Part of the external female genitals at the upper part of the vaginal entrance.
Coitus	Fucking, balling, screwing	Sexual intercourse where the penis is placed in the vagina.
Conception		The fertilization of the egg by a sperm (The beginning of pregnancy)
Condom	Rubber	A thin rubber sheath placed over the penis.
Corona		The rim between the glans and the shaft of the penis.
Cunnilingus	Eat pussy, going down	Licking the female genitals.
Desire	Horny	Sexual interest, appetite, anticipation.
Detumescence	Going soft	Return to the flaccid state when the blood leaves the erectile tissue of the penis.
Dyspareunia		Painful intercourse.
Ejaculation	To come, shoot, explode	The expulsion of semen from the penis during orgasm.

Epididymis		Tubes attached to the testes storing mature sperm.
Erection	Hard on, boner	The enlargement and stiffening of the penis (tumescence) as the erectile tissue is engorged with blood caused by sexual excitement.
Erotic	Hot to trot	Sexually stimulating.
Estrogen		Female sex hormone produced in the ovaries.
Excitement phase	Turned on	A stage in the sexual response cycle.
Fallopian tubes	Plumbing	The tube extending from the ovaries to the uterus to carry the eggs.
Fellatio	Blow job, cock sucker	Licking or sucking the penis.
Flaccid	Limp dick	The unaroused state of the penis.
Foreplay	Petting	Caressing.
Foreskin		The fold of skin covering the glans of the uncircumcised penis.
Frigid	Ice bag, cold	A woman who is sexually unresponsive or unable to have an orgasm.

Genitals	Dick, pussy, cunt, snatch, balls, nuts	The external and internal sexual organs or reproductive organs of men and women.
Gender identity		Psychological: the sense of maleness or femaleness.
Glans clitoris	Clit	The head of the clitoris.
Glans penis	Head	The head of the penis.
Gonads	Balls, family jewels	The testes or ovaries.
Heterosexual	Straight	One who is attracted sexually to the other sex.
Homosexual	Fag, homo, queer, fairy	One who is attracted sexually to persons of the same sex. Women are also called lesbians.
Hymen	Cherry	The thin membrane partially covering the vaginal opening.
Impotence	Can't get it up	Inability to have an erection.
Incest	Mother fucker	Sexual contact between relatives.
Intromission		Inserting the penis in the vagina.
Labia Majora	Lips, muff	The outer lips of the vulva.

Labia Minora		The inner lips lying between the outer lips.
Lesbian	Butch, dyke	A female homosexual.
Libido		A term referring to sex drive/desire.
Lubrication		Glandular secretion in the vagina.
Masturbation	Jerk off, hand job, beat your meat	Sexual self-stimulation of the genitals, usually by hand or a mechanical device.
Menopause		The gradual cessation of menstruation in woman.
Menstruation	Bleeding, period, the curse	The monthly discharge of blood from the uterus.
Mon pubis	Beaver, pussy	Fatty tissue under the female pubic hair.
Nocturnal emission	Wet dream	Ejaculation of semen during sleep.
Oral-genital sex	69, getting down	Cunnilingus or fellatio where the mouth stimulates the genitals
Orgasm	To come	Muscular contractions or intense sensations that is the climax of sexual pleasure followed by male

		ejaculation and relief of conjestion in the female pelvic area.
Ovary		The female reproductive gland which produces eggs and sex hormones.
Penis	Prick, dick	The external male sex organ consisting of erectile tissue and the glans.
Perversion		A deviation from accepted sexual norms: sadism, transvestism, voyeurism and zoophilia.
Petting	Feeling up	Intimate touching and close physical contact.
Phallus	Pecker, peter	Penis.
Plateau phase		The third stage of sexual arousal which follows desire and excitement, prior to orgasm.
Positions		Various positions partners can take during coitus.
Potent		Male's sexual ability to have an erection.

Premature ejaculation	Fast on the draw	When the man ejaculates sooner than desired.
Prepuce		The foreskin which covers the glans.
Prophylactic		Condom.
Pudendum	Beaver, pussy	Female external genitals, i.e., labia majora, clitoris, and the pubic area.
Rape		Forced coitus, usually by a man threatening a woman against her will.
Refractory period		The stage immediately after orgasm.
Resolution phase		The last phase of human sexual response when sexual tensions diminish and the body returns to an unaroused state.
Retarded ejaculation		The male is unable to ejaculate even though he has an erection.
Retrograde ejaculation		The male ejaculates internally and the semen goes to the urinary bladder.
Rhythm method	Russian roulette	Birth control method consisting

		of sexual abstinence during the woman's fertile period.
Scrotum	Ball bag	The pouch that contains the testes.
Semen	Come juice	The fluid containing male sperm that is ejaculated.
Seminal fluid		The liquid part of the semen.
Sensate focus exercise		Exercises to arouse sexual response.
Sex flush		Deepening of skin color during sexual arousal.
Sexism	Male chauvinist, pig	A double standard to stereotype in order to gain social advantage.
Sexual dysfunction		A problem with sexual response causing distress, i.e., unable to get an erection or unable to reach a climax.
Sexual identity		The person's sense of who he or she is and sexual attraction.
Sexual intercourse	Fucking, balling, screwing	Physical contact between a man and a woman where the penis enters the vagina.

Sexual response cycle		Five stages: desire, excitement, plateau, orgasm, and resolution.
Sexuality	Turn on	Physical and emotional expression of closeness, warmth, intimacy, tenderness, and sexual pleasure.
SIECUS		Sex Information and Education Council of the United States, 84 Fifth Avenue, N.Y., N.Y. 10011
Sperm		The male reproductive cell which fertilizes the egg.
Statutory rape	Jail bait	Sexual intercourse with a male or female under the age of legal consent.
Sterile		Infertile; unable to produce children.
Tactile		The sense of touch.
Tampon	Rag	A plug of absorbent material placed in the vagina to absorb menstrual flow.
Testes	Balls, nuts	The male glands located in the scrotum used for producing sperm and hormones.

Testosterone		The male sex hormone produced by the testicles.
Transsexual		A person who feels trapped in the body of a different gender and desires a sex change.
Transvestite	Drag queen	Person who receives sexual gratification by wearing the clothes of the other sex.
Tumescence		Swelling of the organs with fluid.
Urethra		Canal through which urine flows from the bladder. The male canal is used for the passage of semen.
Uterus		Muscular organ at the end of the vagina.
Vagina	Cunt, pussy	The female organ extending from the vulva to the uterus.
Vaginismus		Involuntary spasmatic contraction of the puboccygeal muscles preventing penis insertion.
Vaginitis		Inflammation of the vagina.

Vas deferens

The duct which conveys sperm from the testes to the ejaculatory duct.

Vasectomy

A contraceptive procedure in which the vas deferens is cut/tied preventing the passage of sperm.

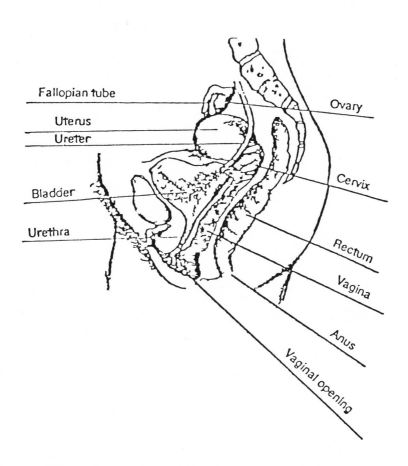

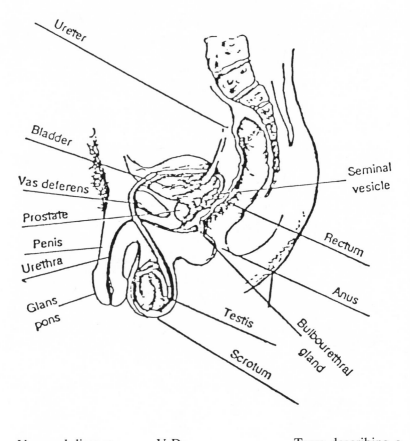

Venereal disease	V.D.	Term describing a number of contagious diseases contracted primarily through sexual intercourse.
Virgin	Inexperienced	A man or woman who has never participated in sexual intercourse.
Vulva	Beaver, pussy	Pudendum.
Zoophilia		Receiving sexual gratification from animals.

Appendix: Resources

The following are texts in alcoholism and sexuality and/or basic to the sex therapy field. This list is intended to provide recommended readings for further study. It is not an exhaustive list of materials in alcohol and sexuality. (See O'Farrell.)

Books/Pamphlets

Annon, J.S. *The Behavioral Treatment of Sexual Problems*, Vol. 1 & 2. Hawaii: Enabling Systems, 1975–1976.

Barbach, L. *For Each Other*. N.Y.: Anchor Press, 1982.

Edelwich, J. and Brodsky, A. *Sexual Dilemmas for the Helping Professional*. N.Y.: Brunner/Mazel, 1982.

Fleit, L. *Alcohol & Sexuality*. Virginia: H/P Publishing Company, 1979.

Gonsiorek, J.C. (ed.), *Homosexuality & Psychotherapy*. N.Y.: Haworth Press, 1982.

Hartman, C., Quinn, J., and Young, B. *Sexual Expression: A Manual for Trainers*. N.Y.: Human Sciences Press, 1981.

Kaplan, H.S., *The New Sex Therapy*. N.Y.: Brunner/Mazel, 1974.

Kaplan, H.S., *The Evaluation of Sexual Disorders*. N.Y.: Brunner/Mazel, 1983.

Lieblum, S.R. and Pervin, L.A. (eds.) *Principles and Practice of Sex Therapy*. N.Y.: Guilford Press, 1980.

Masters, W.H. and Johnson, V.E. *Human Sexual Response*. Boston: Little, Brown & Co., 1966.

Masters, W.H. and Johnson, V.E. *Human Sexual Inadequacy*. Boston: Little, Brown & Co., 1970.

Masters, W.H., Johnson, V.E. and Kolodny, R.C. *Ethereal Issues in Sex Therapy and Research*. Boston: Little, Brown & Co., 1977

O'Farrell, T.J. and Weyand, C.A. *Alcohol & Sexuality: An Annotated Bibliography on Alcohol Use, Alcoholism & Human Sexual Behavior*. Arizona: Oryx Press, 1983.

Smith, D.E. and Buxton, M.E. "Sexological Aspects of Substance Use & Abuse", *Journal of Psychoactive Drugs*, Vol. 14, #1–2, January–June, 1982.
Weinberg, J.R. *Sex & Recovery*. Minneapolis: Recovery Press, 1977.

Journals

Archives of Sexual Behavior
Plenum Publications
233 Spring Street
New York, New York 10013

Journal of Homosexuality
The Haworth Press
28 East 22nd Street
New York, New York 10010

Journal of Marital and Family Therapy
American Association of Marriage & Family Therapy
924 West 9th Street
Upland, California 91786

Journal of Sex & Marital Therapy
Human Sciences Press
72 Fifth Avenue
New York, New York 10011

Journal of Sex Education & Therapy
American Association of Sex Educators, Counselors & Therapists
600 Maryland Ave., S.W.
Washington, D.C. 20024

Medical Aspects of Human Sexuality
Hospital Publications
360 Lexington Avenue
New York, New York 10017

Sexual Medicine Today (Monthly)
International Medical News Service, Inc.
600 New Hampshire Avenue, N.W. — Suite 405
Washington, D.C. 20037

SIECUS Report (Bimonthly)
Behavioral Publications
72 Fifth Avenue
New York, New York 10011

Newsletters

AASECT Newsletter (Quarterly)
American Association of Sex Educators, Counselors and Therapists
2000 N Street, N.W. — Suite 110
Washington, D.C. 20036

MJI Newsletter (Quarterly)
Masters & Johnson Institute
4910 Forest Park Boulevard
St. Louis, Missouri 63108

Organizations in Human Sexuality and Related Fields

American Association of Marriage and Family Counselors
1717 K Street, N.W. - Suite 407
Washington, D.C. 20006

American Association of Sex Educators, Counselors and Therapists (AASECT)
2000 N Street, N.W. - Suite 110
Washington, D.C. 20036

International Academy of Sex Research
c/o Dr. Richard Green
Department of Psychiatry and Behavioral Sciences
Health Sciences Center
School of Medicine - SUNY
Stony Brook, New York 11790

United States Consortium for Sexology
3200 West Market Street - Suite 104
Akron, Ohio 44313

National Council on Family Relations
1219 University Avenue, S.E.
Minneapolis, Minnesota 55411

Planned Parenthood
810 Seventh Avenue
New York, New York 10019

Sex Information and Education Council of U.S. (SIECUS)
80 Fifth Avenue - Suite 801–802
New York, New York 10011

Society for Sex Therapy and Research (SSTAR)
c/o Dr. Alexander Levay
4 East 98th Street
New York, New York 10028

Society for the Scientific Study of Sex
208 Daffodil Road
Glen Burnie, Maryland 21061

Training Aids and Programs in Human Sexuality/Alcoholism

AASECT
2000 N. Street, N.W. - Suite 110
Washington, D.C. 20036

Chemical Dependency & Family Intimacy
Program in Human Sexuality
Department of Family Practice & Community Health
Medical School, University of Minnesota
2630 University Ave., S.E.
Minneapolis, Minnesota 55414

Hazelden
Box 176
Center City, Minnesota 55012

Institute for Integral Development
Post Office Box 2172
Colorado Springs, Colorado 80901

International Council of Sex Research & Parenthood
American University
5010 Wisconsin Avenue, N.W. - Suite 304
Washington, D.C. 20016

Johnson Institute
10700 Olson Memorial Highway
Minneapolis, Minnesota 55441

Masters & Johnson Institute
24 South Kings Highway
St. Louis, Missouri 63108

Patuxent Seminars
5999 Harpers Farm Road
Columbia, Maryland 21044

RAJ Publications
Post Office Box 18599
Denver, Colorado 80218

Shore, David. *Educational and Training Opportunities in Sexology, A Resource Manual*, 1979. Curie, c/o Sullivan House, 1525 East 53rd Street, Chicago, Illinois 60615.

Audiovisual Reviews

The *Journal of Sex and Marital Therapy* has monthly audiovisual reviews.

Daniel, R.S. *Human Sexuality Methods and Materials for the Educator, Family Life and Health Professionals: Annotated Guide to the Audiovisual.* Bree, California: Heuristicus Publishing Company, 1979.

Sex Information Council of U.S. *Film Resources for Sex Education.* Human Sciences Press, 1975.

Singer, Laura. *Sex Education on Film: A Guide to Visual Aids and Programs.* New York: Teachers' College Press.